Stroke

American Academy of Neurology Press
Quality of Life Guides

Austin J. Sumner, MD
Series Editor

Alzheimer's Disease
Paul Dash, MD and Nicole Villemarette-Pittman, PhD
2005

Amyotrophic Lateral Sclerosis
Robert G. Miller, MD, Deborah Gelinas, MD,
and Patricia O'Connor, RN
2005

Migraine and Other Headaches
William B. Young, MD and Stephen D. Silberstein, MD
2004

Stroke
Louis R. Caplan, MD
2005

Stroke

LOUIS R. CAPLAN, MD
Professor of Neurology
Harvard Medical School
and
Chief, Division of Cerebrovascular Disease
Beth Israel Deaconess Medical Center
Boston, Massachusetts

AUSTIN J. SUMNER, MD
Series Editor

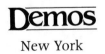

New York

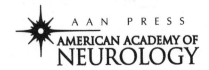

AAN PRESS
AMERICAN ACADEMY OF
NEUROLOGY

Demos Medical Publishing, LLC, 368 Park Avenue South, New York, New York 10016

Uses for products within this text may include those not currently approved by the FDA. For more information on the products, please see full prescribing information.

Library of Congress Cataloging-in-Publication Data
Caplan, Louis R.
   Stroke / Louis R. Caplan. — 1st
         p. cm. — (AAN Press quality of life guide)
   Includes bibliographical references and index.
   ISBN 1-932603-14-X
   1. Cerebrovascular disease—Popular works. I. Title. II. Series.
   RC388.5.C3297   2006
   616.8'1—dc22

                                        2005023147

Made in the United States of America

Copyeditor: Jessica Bryan
Typesetting: Patricia Wallenburg
Indexing: Joann Woy
Printer: The Maple-Vail Book Manufacturing Group

Contents

Contents

About the AAN Press
Quality of Life Guides

IN THE SPIRIT OF THE DOCTOR–PATIENT PARTNERSHIP

THE BETTER-INFORMED PATIENT is often able to play a vital role in his or her own care. This is especially the case with neurologic disorders, for which effective management of disease can be promoted—indeed, *enhanced*—through patient education and involvement.

In the spirit of the partnership-in-care between physicians and patients, the American Academy of Neurology Press is pleased to produce a series of "Quality of Life" guides on an array of diseases and ailments that affect the brain and central nervous system. The series, produced in partnership with Demos Medical Publishing, answers a number of basic and important questions faced by patients and their families.

Additionally, the authors, most of whom are physicians, and all of whom are experts in the areas in which they write, provide a detailed discussion of the disorder, its causes, and the course it may follow. You also find strategies for coping with the disorder and handling a number of nonmedical issues.

The result: As a reader, you will be able to develop a framework for understanding the disease and become better prepared to manage the life changes associated with it.

ABOUT THE AMERICAN ACADEMY OF NEUROLOGY (AAN)

The American Academy of Neurology is the premier organization for neurologists worldwide. In addition to support of educational and scientific advances, the AAN—along with its sister organization, the AAN Foundation—is a strong advocate of public education and a leading supporter of research for breakthroughs in neurologic patient care.

More information on the activities of the AAN is available on our website, www.aan.com. For a better understanding of common disorders of the brain, as well as to learn about people living with these disorders, please turn to the AAN Foundation's website, www.thebrainmatters.org.

ABOUT NEUROLOGY AND NEUROLOGISTS

Neurology is the medical specialty associated with disorders of the brain and central nervous system. Neurologists are medical doctors with specialized training in the diagnosis, treatment, and management of patients suffering from neurologic disease.

Austin J. Sumner, MD
Series Editor
AAN Press Quality of Life Guides

Foreword

STROKE IS COMMON. Stroke can be tragic. The tragedy of major stroke can in some instances be prevented. In any case, it must be understood, and at least made manageable if not overcome. As a health problem, the conditions that affect the blood supply to the brain place a huge burden on the affected individual, the family, and society. In its extreme, stroke is the condition that in a split second can change the very essence of who a person is by drastically altering brain function. In its less destructive manifestation, it affects brain function to produce the most curious behaviors. In this book, Dr. Louis Caplan lays open the mysteries and deals with the realities of stroke in terms that resonate with a reader who has suffered a stroke or known a friend or family member affected by stroke.

Taken in its entirety, stroke seems complicated. However, the complexity relates to the wide variety of stroke types and the parts of brain affected. In fact, an individual stroke and its effect on an individual can be readily understood. Dr. Caplan masterfully conveys the key features that underlie the common stroke types using individual examples. Many of the messages in these case studies are generalizable but he also goes to considerable length to explain the panoply of stroke as well. Since stroke affects particular brain regions, the description of brain dysfunction that follows stroke offers a way to understand the compartmentalization of brain function. In this book, the relationship between what the patient experiences and what brain area is affected is carefully laid out.

The figures are especially useful in projecting the take-home point. This is often what is most difficult for the lay person to understand but is the very foundation of stroke neurology, of which Dr. Caplan is the leading figure.

To the patient and family, the testing and treatment decisions that come so quickly can seem very confusing. For the stroke physician, they are like second nature. Often the physician assumes incorrectly that his logic is obvious to the patient. In these pages, Dr. Caplan thinks through the patient's admission to the hospital, to discharge and rehabilitation, and then home with a prevention plan. He explains each step along the way, and this makes the book a very useful guide. Which medications are prescribed for what reason? Why the many different brain imaging studies? What life style changes can decrease stroke risk? These are the key practical questions that are addressed in this jewel written by a master of the craft of stroke neurology. Dr. Caplan's clinical insights and closeness to the human condition make the book useful and interesting. His direct writing style makes it easy to read and the reader can easily comprehend what otherwise seems so mysterious.

Walter J. Koroshetz, MD
Department of Neurology
Harvard Medical School
Cambridge, MA

Preface

"Knowledge is power."

Francis Bacon

MEDICAL CARE in the twenty-first century has become more complex than at any time in the past. Insurance companies and those who pay for medical care, hospitals, and doctors have created many rules that complicate entry into the medical system and sometimes make it difficult for patients to receive the medical care they need and deserve. Patients and their loved ones face more barriers and hassles than in the past.

Good medical care requires an effective partnership between doctors and patients and their loved ones. In order for individuals to become good consumers and to press for the best medical care, they need to understand the functions of their bodies and the diseases and risks for diseases they are likely to develop as they age. The Internet, and publications aimed at patients and potential patients have greatly proliferated. The public has been deluged with information. Some of the information is too complicated to be easily understood, some of the information is wrong, and some media communications are motivated by marketing strategies aimed at getting people to buy a medicine or to undergo a procedure.

It is especially important for individuals to learn about neurologic diseases. The brain and nervous system are complicated.

Neurologic diseases are often very serious. Non-neurologists are often not fully prepared to diagnose and treat neurologic problems. Stroke is especially important since it has the potential to cause an important life-long disability. Stroke often develops quickly, so individuals need to be prepared for rapid action.

Prevention of stroke is much more likely to have a major impact on the health and welfare of the population than even the most effective treatment after stroke has occurred. For this important reason, much effort is aimed at identifying and modifying whenever possible risk factors for cerebrovascular disease.

Surveys of the public have shown:

- Nearly half of those surveyed were unable to name any early warning signs of stroke; those who did answer often gave incorrect responses.
- Most were not aware that stroke is among the three major causes of death in the United States.
- In answer to the question, "A stroke occurs when the blood supply is cut off to what part of the body?" one third of individuals did not select the brain from the choices of "heart," "brain," "don't know," and "other."
- Some (about 7%) thought that arthritis was a major cause of stroke.
- Only 44% identified weakness or loss of feeling in one arm or leg as a symptom of stroke, as opposed to heart attack.
- Those surveyed overestimated the proportion of stroke patients who become permanently disabled or who require institutionalization after stroke.

A recent report described the results of a structured interview with open-ended questions given to patients in the emergency room at the University of Cincinnati Medical Center during the first 48 hours after they were admitted to the hospital with possible strokes. Among these 163 patients, 63 (39%) did not know a single symptom or sign of stroke. One-sided weakness (26%) and numbness (22%) were the most often mentioned symptoms. Patients over 65 years of age were less knowledgeable than younger patients.

The aim of this book is to try to narrow the information gap between doctors and the public about stroke. I hope to teach about stroke and to do so in as simple a manner as possible. Because pictures are often better than words, I have liberally sprinkled illustrations throughout the book. If this book helps in even a small way to allow some strokes to be prevented, and others to be treated more effectively, it will have met its goal.

Louis R. Caplan, MD
Boston, MA
Fall 2005

Acknowledgments

No project such as this can be carried out by only one individual. I have many to thank and acknowledge. Steve Moskowitz skillfully provided clear illustrations. Dr. Walter Koroshetz, a trusted colleague at the Massachusetts General Hospital and Harvard Medical School, thoroughly reviewed the manuscript and made very helpful suggestions that I have incorporated into the book. Jessica Bryan made editorial suggestions to help make the text more understandable to readers. Cleo Hutton, a stroke hero and a co-author of mine of a previously published book about stroke, provided helpful tips for patients and their caregivers. Dorothy Northrop, a very experienced medical social worker, has contributed her advice on to how to deal with insurers and insurance issues.

Edith Barry and Dr. Diana M. Schneider at Demos Medical Publishing oversaw all aspects of the book's publication. The American Academy of Neurology (AAN) sponsored this book as part of their series of publications aimed at public education. Dr. Austin Sumner deserves thanks for asking me to create this book and for shepherding it for the AAN.

Most of all, I thank my patients and their families and caregivers who have taught me during more than 40 years so much about their medical conditions and about dealing with infirmities. Their insights and courage have been important inspirations for me. I hope and pray that this book will, in some small measure, help future stroke patients so that past stroke patients will not have suffered completely in vain.

Stroke

CHAPTER 1

Introduction: Why Is Stroke So Important?

"It was then that it happened. To my shock and incredulity, I could not speak. That is, I could utter nothing intelligible. All that would come from my lips was the sound *ab*, which I repeated again and again.... Then as I watched it, the telephone handpiece slid slowly from my grasp, and I, in turn, slid slowly from my chair and landed on the floor behind the desk.... At 5:15 in that January dusk I had been a person; now at 6:45 I was a case. But I found it easy to accept my altered condition. I felt like a case."

Eric Hodgins
Episode: Report on the Accident Inside My Skull

EFFECT OF STROKES ON INDIVIDUALS

WHEN SPEAKERS TRY TO IMPRESS their audiences and their readers on the importance of stroke, they usually quote numbers and statistics. But, truly, the most important aspect of stroke is its effect on the individual who develops a stroke. What is more frightening and devastating than to suddenly become unable to speak, understand the speech of others, move an arm or leg, stand, walk, balance, hear, see, read, feel, write, or remember? Loss of function is often instantaneous and totally unanticipated. The first common term for stroke, *apoplexy*, in Greek lit-

> The most important aspect of stroke is its effect on the individual who develops a stroke.

1

erally meant "struck suddenly with violence." The word *stroke* refers to being suddenly stricken. Loss of brain function can be dehumanizing, and often makes individuals dependent on others for ordinary daily activities. The brain is without question the most important organ in the human body. It is responsible for our movements, feelings, moods, thoughts, and perceptions, and it enables our unique personal characteristics, abilities and failings, intelligence, feelings, and our personalities. Our brains make us what we are. The loss of any brain function diminishes the *person* in us. In surveys that ask individuals about their worse health fears, most people rate cancer and stroke at the top of their lists. People worry about the pain of cancer. They fear losing their mental and physical functions, and becoming dependent on others if they were to have a stroke. Everyone wants to exit this life with their capabilities and mind intact, despite the inevitable aging of their bodies.

The quote at the beginning of this chapter was written by Eric Hodgins, the author of the popular best seller *Mr. Blandings Builds His Dream House*. In Hodgins's later book, *Episode: Report on the Accident Inside My Skull*, he describes exactly what it felt like to be suddenly deprived of speech and the movement of his right limbs. He changed from a highly functioning human being in one moment to a helpless, dumb invalid, "a case," in the next instant. Imagine an articulate author dependent for his livelihood on his use of language becoming totally unable to speak or write.

THE COMPLEXITY OF STROKE

Stroke is a complicated condition having many different causes and very different effects on individuals. Loss of function may be temporary or permanent, slight or devastating. Some functions may improve, while others do not. Readers will better understand stroke, as explained in this book, by following the stories of the four stroke patients referred to throughout the book. Their symptoms, stroke risk factors, the causes of their strokes, their evaluations and treatments, and the effects that their strokes had on themselves and their families and environment will be described. The four patients are:

Robert H., a 68-year-old retired engineer who lives with his wife. His three children are married and are no longer living at home. He has had many health problems during the past. His blood pressure was discovered to be high 20 years ago. He was given a number of different pills, but his high blood pressure has remained a problem. Ten years ago, he had a heart attack and had to have heart surgery on his coronary arteries. For the past few years, he has had pain in the right calf of his leg when he walks. His doctors told him that an artery to that leg was narrowed. Similar blood pressure and heart problems had led to his father dying at age 51. His brother also had hypertension and had several heart attacks. One sister had a stroke.

One day at work, he noticed that his left hand and arm felt numb, and he could not hold objects in this hand. The weakness and numbness lasted about 15 minutes. He assumed that he had leaned on the hand. Two days later, shortly after he awakened in the morning, his left face and hand felt numb and tingly for about 5 minutes. That same day, in the afternoon, a shade seemed to come over his right eye and he could not see from that eye for about a minute. These symptoms worried him, and he scheduled appointments with his eye doctor and primary physician. Two days later, in the morning before he had seen either doctor, he fell on the floor when he attempted to get out of bed. His wife heard the fall and rushed to him. She recognized that his left limbs did not move, but he seemed unaware of the nature of the problem. She called an ambulance and rushed him to the emergency room of the hospital.

Claire H., a 29-year-old woman who lives in Boston with her family, took a day trip with her husband and four young children to visit her parents in New York. It was a summer day and the weather and car were very hot. The day was rather hectic, and they had nothing to eat or drink after 2:00 P.M. The family piled into the car at about 5 P.M. for the long trip back to Boston in heavy traffic. The children were restless and irritable, and squabbled nearly continuously in the back of the station wagon. Claire had to kneel on her seat in the front of the car and face backward to try and maintain peace.

When they arrived home, Claire and her husband quickly put the exhausted kids to bed, had a snack and a drink, and also went to bed.

Claire suddenly became unable to speak while having intercourse. Her husband realized that her right limbs had become weak, and he rushed her to the hospital. She began to move her right leg on the way there. She could talk, but did not seem to understand everything that he said. She used some wrong and nonexistent words.

Tom M., a 41-year-old single man, became ill at work. He was a longshoreman and his job was physically demanding. While straining to lift some heavy cargo, he felt dizzy and lurched to his left. He staggered and seemed "drunk" to his co-workers. Several minutes later, he vomited and complained that he had developed a bad headache in the back of his head and in his left neck and shoulder.

Tom had been healthy in the past, but admitted to drinking wine rather heavily. He did not visit doctors regularly. When checked by the company doctor 4 years previously, he had been told that his blood pressure was "a bit high," and that it needed to be rechecked, but he had not followed through.

Sam J. was a 73-year-old man. He had been an accountant, but was now retired. He was a widower and lived alone. His children, who lived in another city, called and visited often. He had a recent onset of atrial fibrillation. Sam had always been healthy, but recently he had noted periods when his heart did not beat regularly. Sometimes when this happened, he became slightly short of breath. He did not have hypertension or diabetes and did not smoke. He was relatively sedentary and did not want to exercise. These short bouts of fast, irregular heartbeats worried him, and he made an appointment with his doctor. Before Sam could schedule a doctor's visit, one afternoon he suddenly realized that his right hand and leg had become weak. He felt tingling over the entire right side of his body, including his face.

THE NUMBERS

Stroke is and has been the third leading cause of death in most countries around the world for a very long time. Only heart disease and cancer are more significant killers. Strokes cause more prolonged disability than any other medical condition. Survivors of strokes are often unable to return

Stroke is the third leading cause of death in most countries around the world.

to work or assume their former effectiveness as spouses, parents, friends, and active participants in their communities. The economic, social, and psychologic costs of stroke are enormous. The direct expense of stroke in the United States is estimated at more than 40 billion dollars each year.

In the United States alone, nearly 750,000 individuals will have a stroke, and 150,000 die from stroke each year (90,000 women and 60,000 men). Someone has a stroke every 45 seconds, and every 3.1 minutes, someone dies of a stroke. There are about 2 million stroke survivors living in the United States at any one time. Stroke affects three times as many women as breast cancer, yet receives much less attention from women's health organizations. In China, about 1.5 million people die each year because of stroke. Despite its importance, stroke research gets much less funding than heart disease, cancer, diabetes, and AIDS. Figure 1-1 shows the relative spending on research for these diseases in 1994 and 1996.

Although strokes are much more common in people over 65, and many people believe that strokes only happen to old folks, strokes can occur at any age, including infancy, childhood, adolescence, and early adulthood. During the last 35 years, I have taken care of over 200 patients who have had strokes before their 40th birthday. There are now several medical books devoted entirely to discussions of strokes in the young. Stroke can happen to anyone. Stroke can happen to you!

STROKES IN HISTORY

The history of the world has undoubtedly been greatly affected by stroke. Many important leaders in science, art, medicine, and politics have had their productivity cut prematurely short by stroke. Louis Pasteur, the great French scientist whose discoveries led to the vaccines that prevent smallpox, had a stroke at age 46 that caused left-sided

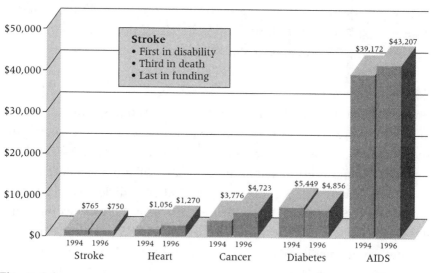

Figure 1-1

Research funding during 1994 and 1996 comparing dollars spent for with those spent for heart disease, cancer, diabetes, and AIDS.

paralysis. In spite of this stroke, he continued to make important advances until additional strokes further impaired his ability to function at age 65. Marcello Malpighi, one of the first individuals to describe the biologic characteristics of the small blood vessels and capillaries, and

> The history of the world has undoubtedly been greatly affected by stroke.

who wrote about the anatomy of the lungs, kidneys, and spleen as seen under a microscope, died of a stroke that had paralyzed his right arm and leg.

Two very important political leaders during the early twentieth century, Vladimir Lenin and Woodrow Wilson, had intellectual impairments related to stroke while they were at the helm of their respective countries during critical times in history. Lenin, at age 52, had a sudden onset of slurred speech and right-sided paralysis. An observer noted that his words were often slurred as he spoke, and he paused several times as if he had lost the thread of his argument. Woodrow Wilson, President of the United States and the architect of the League of Nations during the first quarter of the twentieth century, had a series of small strokes that left him with difficulty speaking and swallowing, and left arm and leg weakness at a time when he was working hard for world peace and cooperation.

All of the heads of state who met at Yalta and elsewhere to divide up the spheres of influence after World War II—including Franklin Roosevelt (U.S.A.), Winston Churchill (Great Britain), and Josef Stalin (Russia)—had severe cerebrovascular disease and had had multiple strokes by the time of their meetings. Figure 1-2 shows these three leaders at a conference. Roosevelt subsequently died of a fatal stroke resulting from brain hemorrhage after years of severe hypertension. There was no effective treatment for high blood pressure during Roosevelt's time. History might have been very different if the brains of these leaders had not been affected by stroke. Public awareness of stroke increased

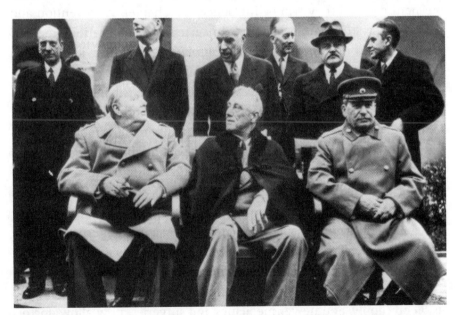

Figure 1-2

Churchill, Roosevelt, and Stalin at a conference in Yalta after World War II. (From Toole J.F. *Cerebrovascular Disorders, Fourth Edition.* New York: Raven Press, 1990.)

dramatically when President Dwight Eisenhower developed a stroke that caused his speech to slur, and when Richard Nixon died after a large acute stroke.

THE PLAN OF THIS STROKE PRIMER

Henry Fielding, the nineteenth century writer and author of the popular book *Tom Jones*, likened an author to a host who has invited special guests to his home for a formal dinner. The host prepares his guests for each course by describing what they are about to eat. Similarly, an author should let readers know what is to come and prepare them for the material that will be set before them.

This introduction emphasizes the importance of stroke both in general and to individuals. The second chapter defines stroke and explains the different mechanisms of stroke and how they cause brain injury. Various medical conditions and risk factors underlie the various stroke mechanisms, and they will be introduced in Chapter 3. Prevention and treatment of strokes is based on management of the various medical conditions and risk factors that cause stroke. Chapter 4 reviews various things that patients and doctors can do to prevent stroke.

In order to understand the symptoms of stroke (Chapter 7), evaluation of patients who have strokes or are at risk of stroke (Chapter 8), and treatment of stroke patients (Chapter 9), it is necessary to learn something about how the brain functions (Chapter 5), and the location and nature of the blood vessels that supply the brain with blood (Chapter 6).

The remaining chapters discuss the complications that sometimes develop after strokes (Chapter 10), disabilities and handicaps that may remain after a stroke (Chapter 11), stroke recovery (Chapter 12), and the effect of one person's stroke on others (Chapter 13). The last chapter provides a look to the future in stroke care and research (Chapter 14).

New and better technologies, able to show images of the brain and its blood supply, and newer medicines and surgeries, now allow doctors to treat stroke patients more successfully than at any time in the past. Much more is known now about stroke prevention, stroke care, and stroke recovery. The future is indeed bright.

CHAPTER 2

What Is a Stroke? What Are the Causes? What Are the Different Kinds of Stroke?

"A sensible man confronted by a sick person would ask himself three simple questions. 'What is wrong with him? How did he get this way? How can I help him?'"

Dr. Mack Lipkin
The Care of Patients

IN ORDER FOR READERS to understand how they can prevent stroke, the conditions doctors look for in order to try and prevent strokes from occurring, how doctors evaluate patients with stroke, and how they treat stroke patients, it is clearly necessary to understand what a stroke is, what causes it, and some of the symptoms. As the quote from Dr Lipkin states, doctors must try to find out what exactly is wrong with someone before they can effectively treat that person. This chapter discusses the different conditions that occur in stroke patients.

WHAT IS A STROKE?

The brain, and every other organ in the body, depends on a constant supply of energy to function normally. Fuel for the brain is carried in the blood. The brain requires more fuel than any other organ in the body. The two main energy sources that the brain uses are sugar and oxygen. Oxygen is carried mainly in the hemoglobin of red blood cells; sugar is carried in the serum of the blood. When a part of the brain does not receive an adequate supply of blood, or when the blood does not carry enough oxygen or sugar, that portion of the brain becomes unable to perform its normal functions. *Stroke* is a term that is used to describe brain injury caused by an abnormality of the blood supply to a part of the brain. The word is derived from the fact that most stroke patients are

> Stroke is a term that is used to describe brain injury caused by an abnormality of the blood supply to a part of the brain.

struck suddenly by blood vessel abnormality, and abnormalities of brain function begin quickly, sometimes within an instant.

Stroke is a very broad term that describes a variety of different types of diseases involving the blood vessels that supply the brain with needed nourishment and fuel. Treatment depends on the type of stroke and the location of the blood vessels involved. Thus, it is very important for treating doctors to determine precisely what caused the vascular and brain injury, and where the abnormalities are located.

WHAT ARE THE DIFFERENT TYPES OF STROKES?

Strokes can be divided into two very broad groups: hemorrhage and ischemia. *Hemorrhage* refers to bleeding inside the skull, either into the brain or into the fluid surrounding the brain. The second major types of stroke are called ischemia, a term that refers to a lack of blood. *Emia* is a suffix that always refers to blood. Hemorrhage and ischemia are polar opposites. Hemorrhage is characterized by too much blood inside the

> Strokes can be divided into two very broad groups: hemorrhage and ischemia.

skull. In ischemia, there is not enough blood supply to allow continued normal functioning of the effected brain tissue. Brain ischemia is much more common than hemorrhage. About four strokes out of every five are ischemic.

Hemorrhage

There are several different subtypes of hemorrhage; they are named for their locations inside of the skull. The brain is surrounded by three membranes; from inside toward the skull they are called: *pia mater, arachnoid,* and *dura mater.* These names come from Latin. *Pia mater* means "soft mother." This inner membrane is thin and covers the brain; it resembles Saran wrap. *Arachnoid* means "like a small insect." This name was given because of the observation that this membrane resembles a spider web. The outer membrane is firm and more substantial than the others and is called *dura mater,* literally meaning "hard mother." These layers are shown in Figure 2-1.

Hemorrhages within the brain substance (inside of the pia mater) are called *intracerebral hemorrhages.* Those between the pia mater and arachnoid are called *subarachnoid hemorrhages.* Hemorrhages outside of

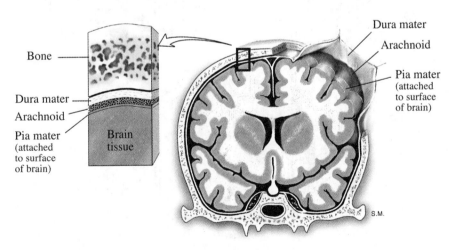

Figure 2-1

The membranes around the brain.

the arachnoid but inside of the dura mater are called *subdural hemorrhages,* and hemorrhages outside of the dura mater but inside of the skull are called *epidural hemorrhages.* These sites of bleeding are shown in Figure 2-2. The different sites of bleeding have different causes.

Bleeding into the brain is referred to as *intracerebral hemorrhage*—intracerebral meaning into the *cerebrum* (another term often used for the brain). Bleeding into the brain results from rupture of small blood vessels—the arterioles and capillaries within the brain substance. The bleeding tears and disconnects vital nerve centers and pathways. Intracerebral hemorrhage is most often caused by uncontrolled *hypertension* (high blood pressure). Other less common causes are listed in Table 2-1. The blood usually oozes into the brain under pressure and forms a localized,

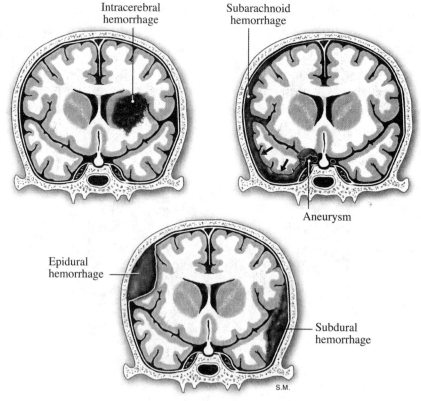

Figure 2-2

Examples of intracerebral, subarachnoid, subdural, and epidural hemorrhages.

Table 2-1 The Most Common Causes and Sites of Hemorrage

Intracerebral hemorrhages
  Hypertension
  Abnormal bleeding functions
    Prescribed anticoagulants such as coumadin
    Low platelet count (thrombocytopenia)
    Bleeding tendencies such as hemophilia
    After receiving thrombolytic drugs
  Vascular malformations
  Amyloid within blood vessels in the brain
  Trauma
  Bleeding into brain tumors and brain infarcts
Subarachnoid hemorrhages
  Arterial aneurysms
  Vascular malformations near the brain surface
  Bleeding tendencies
  Head injury
Subdural hemorrhages
  Trauma
  Bleeding tendencies
Epidural hemorrhages
  Trauma

often round or elliptical blood collection called a *hematoma*. The hematoma separates normal brain structures and interrupts brain pathways, called *tracts*. Hematomas also exert pressure on brain regions adjacent to the collection of blood and can injure these tissues. Large hemorrhages are often fatal because they increase pressure within the skull, squeezing vital regions within the brainstem.

Bleeding into the fluid around the brain is called *subarachnoid* hemorrhage, because the blood collects and stays under the arachnoid membrane that lies over the pia mater. Subarachnoid hemorrhages are usually caused by rupture of an *aneurysm*, a weakened artery with a wall that is ballooned outward. The artery breaks, spilling blood instantly into the spinal fluid that circulates around the brain and spinal cord. The sudden release of blood under high pressure increases the pressure inside the skull and causes severe, sudden-onset headache, often with vomiting. The sudden increase in pressure causes a lapse in brain function, and the patient may stare, drop to his knees, or become confused and unable to remember anything.

Most often, the symptoms in patients with subarachnoid hemorrhage relate to a general decrease in brain function, because usually there is no bleeding into one part of the brain. The decreased function is caused by increased pressure within the skull. In contrast, in patients with intracerebral hemorrhages, the hematoma is localized and causes loss of function related to the area damaged by the local blood collection. For example, if the bleeding occurs into the left cerebral hemisphere, the patient often has weakness and loss of feeling in the right limbs and a loss of normal speech, whereas a hemorrhage into the cerebellum will cause dizziness and a loss of balance.

Tom M., who was introduced in Chapter 1, had an intracerebral hemorrhage into his left cerebellum. Recall that he suddenly became dizzy, staggered, and vomited. He became unable to walk. The cerebellum is specialized for balance, equilibrium, and coordination in walking. Tom's cerebellar hematoma disrupted these important functions. The particular symptoms that patients with intracerebral hemorrhages develop relate to the region of bleeding. They are described as *focal*, that is, related to dysfunction of only one brain region; for example, the left cerebellum in the case of Tom M. The symptoms are diffuse and not localized to one area in subarachnoid hemorrhage.

Subdural and epidural hemorrhages are most often caused by head injuries that tear blood vessels. In subdural hemorrhages, bleeding is usually from veins that lie within the space between the arachnoid membrane and the dura mater. Bleeding most often results in tearing of meningeal arteries in epidural hemorrhages. Often there is an accompanying skull fracture that tears a meningeal artery. Blood accumulates much faster when it issues from arteries than it does when the source is small veins, so that symptoms usually develop soon after head injury in patients with epidural hemorrhages. Bleeding can be slow in subdural hemorrhages, and symptoms of headache and brain dysfunction may be delayed for weeks after the head injury. Subdural hemorrhages may develop in elderly individuals after only minor head injury or even seem to occur spontaneously. Trivial bumps on the head are easily forgotten.

The most common causes of hemorrhages at the various sites are listed in Table 2-1.

The skull forms a closed hard sphere, a fortress around the brain and the surrounding membranes. This fortress can become a prison that limits the exit of blood from within the skull. The closed system means that the bleeding causes pressure to quickly build up and strangle normal tissues by compressing them.

Brain Ischemia

A decrease of blood supply to the brain is called *ischemia*. If the ischemia is prolonged enough, it leads to the death of tissue, which is called *infarction*.

> A decrease of blood supply to the brain is called *ischemia*.

There are three different major categories of brain ischemia, each indicating a different mechanism of blood vessel injury or reason for decreased blood flow. These three categories are often referred to as *thrombosis, embolism,* and *systemic hypoperfusion.* Figure 2-3 illustrates these different mechanisms of ischemia.

These terms are best understood by using an analogy to house plumbing. Suppose that one morning when you turn on the faucet in the bathroom on the second floor no water comes out, or that water only dribbles out. The malfunctioning sink could be due to a local problem, such as rust build-up in the pipe leading to that sink. This type of problem is analogous to *thrombosis,* the term used to describe a local problem involving a blood vessel (artery) that supplies the brain. *Atherosclerosis* is the most common disease that narrows the blood flow channel (lumen) in an artery. When the lumen becomes very narrow, blood flow is severely reduced, causing localized stagnation of the blood column. This change in flow causes the blood to clot, resulting in total occlusion of the artery. Clearly, this is similar to a local problem in one specific pipe, and a plumber would approach the problem by attempting to fix the damaged, blocked pipe. Similarly, treating physicians could treat a narrowed (stenosed) or occluded artery by trying to open it or by

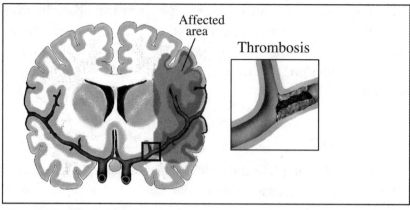

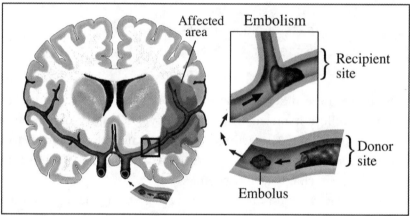

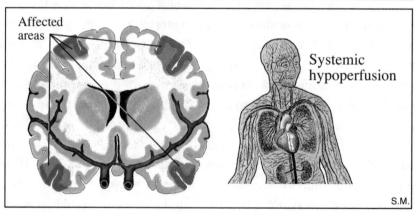

Figure 2-3

The different types of ischemic stroke: thrombosis, embolism, and systemic hypoperfusion.

creating a detour around it. Robert H., who was introduced in Chapter 1, had a stroke due to thrombosis of the right internal carotid artery in his neck. Further chapters will discuss how Robert's doctors were able to show the nature of his problem and how they treated him.

Alternatively, blockage of the pipe to the second floor sink could have been the result of debris in the water system that happened by chance to come to rest in that particular pipe, rather than from a local problem that began within the pipe. An artery within the head or neck that supplies the brain can be blocked by a blood clot or other particulate matter that breaks loose from a downstream site. The source could be from one of three locations: the heart, the aorta (the major artery leading away from the heart), or from one of the major arteries in the neck, which are located before the blocked artery but along the same circulatory pathway. The process of particles breaking loose and blocking a distant artery is referred to as *embolism*. The source of the material is called the *donor site*; the receiving vessel is called the *recipient site*. The material is called an *embolus*; the process of material breaking loose and lodging downstream is called *embolism*. Claire H., who was introduced in Chapter 1, had an embolus that arose in a vein in her leg, passed through her heart, and traveled to the left middle cerebral artery in her head, shutting off blood flow to a portion of her left cerebral hemisphere. This caused her to develop weakness of her right limbs and a speech abnormality. Her evaluation and treatment will be discussed in a later chapter.

Another reason for poor flow in the second floor sink might be a general problem with the water tank, water pump, or water pressure. In this case, the flow of water to all of the sinks and baths in the house would be affected. Simply turning on the faucet in the other sinks in the house will reveal the nature of the problem. In the body, this type of problem is referred to as *systemic hypoperfusion*. Abnormal performance of the heart (pump) could lead to low pressure in the system. Abnormally slow or fast heart rhythms, cardiac arrest, and failure of the heart to pump blood adequately can all lead to diminished blood flow to the head and brain. Another cause of diminished circulatory functions is the lowering of blood pressure and blood flow resulting from an inadequate amount of blood and fluid in the vascular compartment of the body. Bleeding, dehydration, and loss of fluid into body tissues (shock) can all lead to inadequate brain perfusion. This would be akin to having an empty or very low water tank. Figure 2-4 illustrates the mechanisms of this plumbing analogy.

One artery is usually blocked in patients with brain embolism and thrombosis, leading to dysfunction of the part of the brain supplied by that blocked artery. This shows itself by *focal* abnormalities of brain function, such as weakness of the limbs on one half of the body. In this

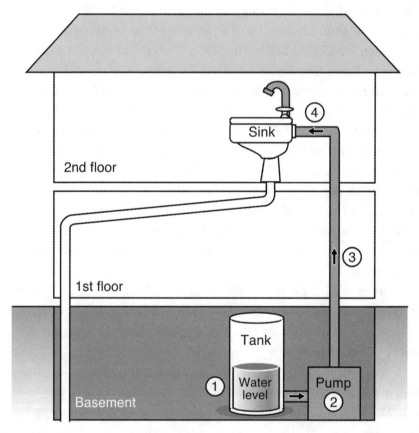

Figure 2-4

Diagram of home plumbing illustrating possible problem areas: (1) insufficient water in the tank; (2) low pump pressure; (3) low water pressure in the pipes; and (4) rust or blockage in a pipe leading direction to the sink.

respect, the abnormalities are similar to those found in patients with local brain hematomas. In contrast, systemic hypoperfusion leads to more diffuse abnormalities such as light-headedness, dizziness, confusion, dimming of vision, and reduced hearing. Patients appear pale and generally weak. These symptoms are caused by a generalized reduction in blood flow, and not to loss of function in one local region of the brain.

The importance of differentiating the types of ischemia is obvious. Returning to the plumbing analogy, a local problem in one pipe (thrombosis) could be potentially fixed by work on that particular pipe. But if the problem is caused by a temporary blockage of that same pipe by loose matter in the system, then removing the blockage in the occluded

> The importance of differentiating the types of ischemia is obvious.

pipe would likely be followed by another pipe being blocked later by the same problem. Somehow the particles must be removed from the system and their subsequent formation should be prevented if possible. If the problem is in the pump, tank, or water pressure work on a single pipe will not be helpful.

Brain ischemia, by definition, refers to an inadequate supply of blood to a part of the brain. Arteries bring sugar, oxygen, and other nutrients necessary for survival to the brain region. An analogy would be a yard with grass or a vegetable garden. If water and sun are inadequate, and the ground does not contain enough nourishment, the grass and vegetables will eventually die. Grass often appears brown before it dies, but watering may restore its normal green color and appearance. Similarly, if the lack of blood flow is brief or relatively minor in degree, there may be temporary loss of function during a brief period of ischemia, but function may return to normal when blood flow is restored. Temporary decreases in blood flow to a part of the brain are often referred to as *transient ischemic attacks* (TIAs). These attacks are caused by temporary blockage of an artery by an embolus that passes, or by temporary inadequacy of blood flow through a narrowed artery.

These temporary attacks indicate that something is wrong with the system and warn of the possibility of a stroke.

Robert H. had several TIAs before his stroke. His left hand and arm went numb in one brief episode. His left face and hand tingled in another attack. These TIA spells indicated a temporary decrease in blood flow to a portion of his right cerebral hemisphere, which controls movement and feeling in his face, arm, and hand. In yet another episode, Robert H. temporarily lost vision in his right eye. This indicated a transient decrease in blood flow to that eye. The right eye and the right cerebral hemisphere are supplied with blood by the right internal carotid artery. These episodes indicated that blood flow was a problem in that artery, but unfortunately Robert H. and his doctors did not attend to this problem, and Robert developed a severe stroke due to total blockage of his right internal carotid artery.

Having discussed the way that abnormalities of blood and blood flow cause brain injury and strokes, the next chapter discusses the types of conditions that damage the structures supplying the brain with blood.

CHAPTER 3

What Are the Medical Conditions that Cause the Blood Vessel and Heart Damage that Lead to Stroke?

"The disorders of the human body and the symptoms indicating them, are as various as the elements of which the body is composed."

Thomas Jefferson
A letter to Dr. Caspar Wistar, June 21, 1807

BLOOD IS PUMPED FROM THE HEART to the aorta, the large artery that first receives blood destined for the brain and other body organs. Several major arteries branch out from the aorta and carry blood to the brain. Abnormalities of the heart, arteries supplying the brain with blood, and of the blood itself are the root causes of brain ischemia and brain hemorrhage, the mechanisms of stroke described in the preceding chapter.

BLOOD VESSELS

In order to understand the various conditions affecting blood vessels, it is necessary to know something of the composition and function of the arteries that bring blood *to* the brain and the veins that drain blood *from* the brain.

Arteries contain three coats, an inner, relatively thin *intima* coat containing an inner membrane called the *endothelium*, a *media* coat that is

21

composed of smooth muscle and elastic and connective tissue, and an outer coat called the *adventitia*. Figure 3-1 shows the different layers within normal arteries. The inner coat, lined by endothelium, forms a barrier between the blood within the center of the artery (lumen) and the wall of the artery. The normal vascular endothelium is ideally suited to prevent blood clotting. The flexibility and the ability for muscle contraction within the medial coat gives the artery the ability to narrow (constrict) or widen (dilate), allowing the artery to change capacity as needed by the organ being supplied with blood.

Arteries bring blood to the brain. Blood is drained away from the brain by veins on the surface of the brain and within the dura mater. Veins have thinner walls and do not have a muscular coat. Clots that form in the veins that drain the brain can lead to increased back pressure and cause hemorrhage into the brain substance. Blood drained from the brain will go into the right side of the heart, then to the lungs, where it will pick up oxygen. The passage of blood to and from the lungs is called the *pulmonary circulation*. Blood goes from the lungs back to the left side of the heart, where it will again be pumped to the aorta and the *systemic circulation*, which goes to the rest of the body.

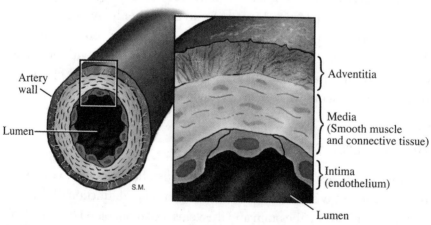

Figure 3-1

Cross-section of a normal artery showing the various coats.

CONDITIONS THAT CAUSE BRAIN ISCHEMIA AND INFARCTION

Atherosclerosis (Arteriosclerosis)

Degenerative changes in the arteries that supply blood to vital organs develop to some extent in all of us if we live long enough. This degeneration is most often referred to as atherosclerosis (*athero* referring to fatty accumulations and *sclerosis* to hardening). Arteriosclerosis (literally "hardening of arteries") is another common term used. This degenera-

> Degenerative changes in the arteries that supply blood to vital organs develop to some extent in all of us if we live long enough.

tion is characterized by the development of plaques on the inside of arteries and wear and tear affecting the wall of the arteries, leading to decreased elasticity and stiffness of the arteries. Atherosclerotic plaques (*atheromas*) develop in the aorta and in the large arteries in the neck and head that supply the brain with blood.

The earliest atherosclerotic abnormalities are called "fatty streaks." They are visible as regions of yellowish discoloration of the intima of the aorta and large and medium-sized systemic and cerebrovascular arteries. Fatty streaks can begin to develop during childhood. The fat comes from fatty substances (lipids) within the blood. The lipid is deposited within and outside of cells, and accumulates along with smooth muscle cells beneath the intima to form the fatty streaks. Later in life, firm (fibrous) plaques develop in the same regions as the fatty streaks. These plaques consist of lipid, smooth muscle, fibrous tissue, connective tissue, white blood cells, and crystals of cholesterol. Some plaques are soft; others are very firm, and may even be calcified.

When atherosclerotic plaques enlarge, they narrow the lumen of the artery and decrease blood flow, which causes changes in the blood stream, often with turbulence. Figure 3-2 shows a large plaque encroaching on the lumen of an artery. The irregular surface of the

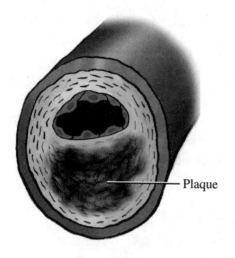

Figure 3-2

Large atherosclerotic plaque
narrowing an artery.

Plaque

plaque attracts small structures within the blood called *platelets*. The platelets stick to each other and form bonds with *fibrin*, a protein formed in the blood from *fibrinogen*. The platelet-fibrin clumps are white, and so they are often called *white clots*. They stick to each other and to the rough regions on the surface of the plaques, as illustrated in Figure 3-3. In addition, cracks in the plaques activate clotting factors in the blood. Red blood cells form a mesh with fibrin. These clots derive their color from the red blood cells, and so they are often called *red clots*.

Atherosclerotic large-artery abnormalities cause ischemia in three major ways: (1) severe luminal narrowing markedly decreases blood flow, leading to brain ischemia in the territory of the compromised artery (*hypoperfusion*); (2) plaques or occlusive *thrombi* mechanically block branches of the main arteries, leading to hypoperfusion in the distribution of these branches of the artery; and (3) propagation and *embolization* of thrombi cause occlusion of distal branches. Emboli can consist of red thrombi, white platelet-fibrin aggregates, or elements of plaques such as cholesterol crystals.

Robert H. had an atherosclerotic plaque in his right internal carotid artery in the neck. Small particles broke off and caused his TIAs when the plaque narrowed the artery. The severe narrowing of the artery slowed blood flow and allowed a red clot to form, which totally occluded the artery. A large part of this red clot broke off and moved into his head, causing his stroke.

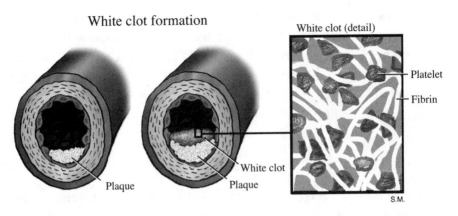

Figure 3-3

Plaque forming in an artery and white platelet-fibrin thrombus attached to the plaque. The boxed illustration shows a white clot as it looks under a microscope.

Several conditions promote and accelerate the development of atherosclerotic plaques, including hypertension, especially if not well controlled, cigarette smoking, high blood cholesterol levels (elevated low density lipoproteins [LDL] and low high density lipoproteins [HDL]), and diabetes, especially if not well controlled. These factors will be discussed in relation to the prevention of stroke in the next chapter.

Hypertension

High blood pressure (hypertension) leads to wear and tear on arteries. Picture again a plumbing situation in which the water pressure is quite high. The pipes and the walls of the pipes might become thinned and rusted with time. Similarly, high blood pressure in the body accelerates the development of atherosclerotic changes in the large arteries of the neck and head. Plaque development is more severe and occurs earlier in life than when blood pressure is normal. Hypertension also leads to

> Hypertension is the single most important risk for brain ischemia and brain hemorrhage.

thickening of the walls of small arteries within the brain. This thickening narrows the lumen of the arteries and can lead to infarcts deep within the brain. Hypertension can also lead to rupture of small arteries within the brain. This will be described in further detail later in this chapter. Hypertension is the single most important risk for brain ischemia and brain hemorrhage.

Arterial Dissection

The term *dissection* refers to a tear in an artery. Sudden movements and stretching, as well as direct injury to an artery, can cause the wall of the artery to tear. Portions of the neck arteries destined to supply the brain are anchored in the neck and where they pass into the skull. Other portions of these arteries are quite mobile and can be stretched and torn. Tears cause bleeding within the arterial wall. The wall swells and may block blood flow. A clot within the arterial wall can be discharged into the lumen of the artery and from there embolize into the brain. Arteries within the skull can also be torn, causing brain infarction or subarachnoid hemorrhage. They are also a significant cause of stroke in children and young adults. Dissections are an important complication of neck manipulation and neck injury. Dissections may develop after seemingly trivial strains such as coughing, vomiting, turning the neck quickly, and extension of the neck in a beauty parlor. Figure 3-4 shows a dissection within an artery.

Fibromuscular Dysplasia (FMD)

This uncommon condition arises in the wall of the artery when there is an excess amount of smooth muscle and connective tissue in the wall. This excess tissue can narrow the arterial lumen. The excess smooth muscle can contract and narrow the lumen. This vasoconstriction can block blood flow to the brain, causing infarction. The vessels are also more vulnerable than normal to strain and dissection. FMD is more common in women. This disorder also can involve the arteries to the kidneys (*renal arteries*), causing hypertension.

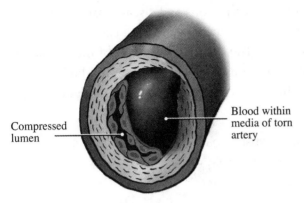

Figure 3-4

A hematoma within the arterial wall caused by dissection of the artery.

Compressed lumen

Blood within media of torn artery

Embolism from the Heart and Aorta

Blood clots and other particles can be released into the blood stream from the heart and aorta. These particles are carried within the flowing blood toward the brain and to other organs, somewhat like a boat being carried vigorously upstream by a rapidly flowing stream. Similarly, in the body, clots and other particles are driven forward within the blood vessels by the force of the contractions of the heart and the blood pressure within the arteries. Arteries become smaller as they reach the organs that they supply, especially after branchings. Depending on their size and makeup, particles can get stuck at branch points and where the arterial passage in which they flow is smaller than the embolic material. Blockage of an artery deprives the brain of blood and nutrition (Figure 3–4). The blockage of the artery might be temporary, because the embolic material can break up and slip through the block point. However, the brain will become infarcted if the blocking lasts long enough. Small emboli cause small infarctions; large emboli may destroy an entire half of the brain. Because important brain functions can require only a small area in the brain to work normally, even small emboli can cause important loss of function. Similar-sized small emboli that reach the lungs, kidneys, and other body organs often cause no symptoms.

A number of different heart conditions and diseases can lead to brain embolism. Understanding of these conditions will be easier if the anatomy of the heart is understood. The heart is the center of the circulatory system; it pumps blood continuously to the various vital body organs, including the brain. The heart is divided after birth into two quite sepa-

> A number of different heart conditions and
> diseases can lead to brain embolism.

rate circulatory systems, one supplying blood to the lungs (pulmonary circulation), and one supplying the brain and the rest of the body (systemic circulation). Each side of the heart has two chambers: an upper chamber called the *atrium*, and a lower chamber called the *ventricle*. Blood returns from the veins of the body into the right side of the heart and enters into its upper chamber, the right atrium. The various body organs have used up the oxygen in this blood, so the returning venous blood is blue. The blood then passes through a valve (called the *tricuspid valve*, because it has three cusps) that lies between the right atrium and the lower muscular chamber, the right ventricle. The right ventricle pumps the blood through a different valve, the *pulmonic valve*, into the main *pulmonary arteries*, which supply the lungs.

The blood is then reinfused with oxygen in the lungs. When it returns to the heart through the pulmonary veins, it is bright pink or red, indicating high oxygen content. The oxygenated blood returning to the heart from the lungs goes into the left side of the heart. It enters the left upper chamber (the left atrium), and then passes through the *mitral valve*, which lies between the left atrium and left ventricle. (The mitral valve derives its name from its similar appearance to a bishop's miter hat.) Next, the left ventricle pumps the oxygenated blood through the *aortic valve* into the *aorta*, the main artery leading to the many systemic artery branches taking oxygen to the tissues. The blood is returned to the right side of the heart for another journey through the lungs after the organs have extracted oxygen.

The valves in the heart make sure that blood goes in the correct direction and not backwards from the ventricles into the *atria* (the two

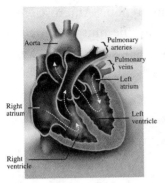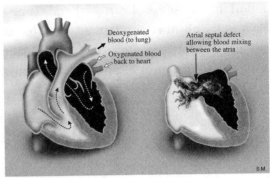

Figure 3-5

The heart, heart valves, and an atrial septal defect.

upper chambers of the heart), or from the pulmonary arteries and aorta back into the ventricles. After the chambers have contracted and expelled their blood contents, the valves close behind the contractions. Figure 3-5 shows the heart and its various chambers, and a defect in the atrial septum.

Atrial Fibrillation

Atrial fibrillation is a very common condition that becomes even more common as people age. About 1 in every 200 individuals has atrial fibrillation. As many as 5% of the people over age 60 may have atrial fibrillation. Atrial fibrillation describes inefficient irregular contractions of the atria, which become dilated, causing blood to pool within them because of the inefficient contractions. This pooling of blood leads to stagnation and the formation of red clots within the atria. These clots can then pass into the ventricles and from there into the aorta and the arteries feeding the brain and other organs.

Myocardial Infarcts

Myocardial infarcts, commonly known as "heart attacks," are another common source of brain embolism. Atherosclerosis, described earlier as a very important cause of brain ischemia and infarction, is also the most important cause of heart ischemia and infarction. Atherosclerotic plaques within the coronary arteries that supply the muscle (*myocardium*) of the heart become blocked with plaques. Blockage of these arteries leads to infarction of portions of heart muscle. Damage to the heart

> Myocardial infarcts, commonly known as "heart attacks," are another common source of brain embolism.

muscle and its inner lining leads to depositing of clots within the interior of the heart. These clots can then be pumped by heart contractions into the aorta and blood stream. Various inflammatory conditions (*myocarditis*) and a variety of other disorders (*myocardiopathies*) that affect the heart muscle can cause poor pumping function, similar to myocardial infarction, thus predisposing a person to forming clots within the heart and later embolizing to the brain.

Valvular Heart Disease

The heart valves are another site of disease that can lead to brain embolism. The valves within the heart serve very important functions. They open to allow blood to flow in the desired direction and then close to prevent blood from flowing back into the previous location. Valve disease can cause hardening of valves, which can impair mobility and narrow the space available for blood to flow. This is called *valvular stenosis*. When a valve fails to close efficiently, allowing backflow, the condition is called *valve insufficiency*.

Rheumatic fever was once the major cause of heart valve inflammation and disease. Although the frequency of rheumatic fever and rheumatic heart disease is decreasing, it is still an important cause of heart disease. This condition often affects the mitral and aortic valves, causing *mitral insufficiency* and *mitral stenosis*. *Aortic stenosis* and *aortic insufficiency* are also common. Some children are born with abnormal heart valves. Aging can also lead to degenerative changes within the valves. One relatively common valve condition that is especially frequent in women is called *mitral valve prolapse*. This means that portions of the mitral valve go backward into the atrium instead of entirely going into the left ventricle. Mucoid material can be deposited within the mitral valve and cause this abnormal functioning. Heart valves can also be damaged by infection. This is usually termed *bacterial endocarditis*. Valve diseases can lead to discharge of a number of different types of particles into the blood stream: white and red blood clots, and pieces of calcium, bacteria, and fibers that collect along the valve. Poorly functioning valves sometimes need to be replaced surgically. Clots can form on artificial valves and become a source of embolism.

Congenital Heart Disease

Some heart problems are congenital, meaning that the defects are present at birth and continue. Some people have holes between their left and right atria or ventricles. These are referred to as *atrial* or *ventricular*

> Some heart problems are congenital.

septal defects. An individual can develop a blood clot (*thrombus*) in a vein somewhere in the body for many reasons, especially in a leg vein. Sitting for a long time in one position, crossing the legs and thereby compressing the veins, abnormal leg veins, and an abnormally increased tendency for blood clotting are just some of the reasons for leg vein thrombosis. When the clot first forms, it can break loose and go to the heart with the returning venous blood. These clots most often go into the right atrium, through the tricuspid valve into the right ventricle, and then through the pulmonary arteries into the lungs. This condition is called *pulmonary embolism*, and it can be very serious. When there is a hole between the two atria, a thrombus formed in the leg veins reaching the right atrium can pass through the hole (*atrial septal defect*) into the left atrium, and then through the mitral valve into the left ventricle. From there the clot goes through the aortic valve into the aorta, and finally

31

into one of its systemic branches. The embolus can cause a brain infarct if it enters one of the arteries to the brain. Defects can cause clots to pass between the two circulations. Strokes caused in this way are called *paradoxical embolism*.

The lungs of babies do not breathe air before birth. During life in the uterus, a hole exists in the wall that separates the babies' left and right atria. This hole allows blood to go from the baby to the mother's circulatory system for oxygenation. This oval shaped hole, which is called the *foramen ovale* (a Latin phrase meaning "oval window"), usually closes at birth. However, it does not fully close in about 30% of individuals.

Claire H. had a paradoxical embolus through a *patent foramen ovale* (PFO). A clot formed in one of her leg veins while she sat backwards in the front seat of the car. This clot traveled to her right atrium during sex, then through the foramen ovale and into her brain, causing her to have a stroke. The clot went into her left cerebral hemisphere, resulting in loss of speech and right-sided limb weakness. Only a very small proportion of individuals with a patent foramen ovale ever have a stroke due to paradoxical embolism.

Disease of the Aorta

The aorta is the largest artery within the body, and the arteries that supply the brain arise from the beginning portion of the aorta within the chest. This part of the aorta, and the aorta within the abdomen, are regions in which atherosclerosis can be quite severe. *Atheromatous plaques* within the aorta in the chest can block arteries to the head. Red and white clots often form on the surface of aortic plaques. These clots, as well as calcium particles and pieces of cholesterol within plaques, can break loose and be carried by the bloodstream into the arteries that feed the brain.

Excess Clotting Resulting from Abnormalities of the Blood

The ability of the blood to clot is a very important defense mechanism. Physical injuries frequently cause the breakage of small blood vessels.

> The ability of the blood to clot is a very
> important defense mechanism.

Components of the blood plug the regions of blood vessel injury, preventing excess bleeding. A deficiency of these blood factors leads to excess bleeding; other conditions lead to excess clotting.

The two most important parts of the body's clotting system are blood platelets and proteins within the blood and blood vessel walls that promote blood clotting. Platelets (also called *thrombocytes*, a term that literally means "clotting cells") are tiny cells that circulate within the blood. When there is a blood vessel injury, and the endothelial lining is broken, platelets circulating in the blood are drawn to the injured region. They adhere to the point of injury and stick together, forming a plug. Clotting is excessive when there are too many platelets (*thrombocytosis*). Dehydration, infections, some medicines, and changes that occur during and just after pregnancy can also promote excessive blood clotting.

Some blood proteins (*antithrombin lll, protein C,* and *protein S*) inhibit the blood from clotting when they are present in normal amounts. When there is a deficiency of one of these substances, usually from birth, then blood clotting will be excessive. There will be an increased tendency for the blood to clot when other blood clotting proteins are excessive; for example, *factors Vll, Vlll,* or *Xll.* Thrombi can develop within blood vessels that have plaques, within apparently normal small blood vessels, and within the veins that drain the brain.

CONDITIONS THAT CAUSE BRAIN AND SUBARACHNOID HEMORRHAGE

Hypertension

Hypertension is the most significant risk factor for bleeding within the brain. Sudden increases in blood pressure severely stress small arteries within the brain and can cause them to break, resulting in hemorrhage into brain substance. Chronic, poorly controlled hypertension also produces wearing down of the walls of the small arteries so that small out-pouchings (*micro-aneurysms*) develop. These outpouchings are not visible grossly, but are seen only through a microscope. The walls of the out-pouchings are thin and can break, especially when exposed to high blood pressure. Occasionally, hypertension can cause the rupture of small arteries on the surface of the brain. Bleeding in this case is sub-arachnoid, into the fluid around the brain.

Uncontrolled hypertension was the cause of Tom's cerebellar hem-orrhage. His blood pressure was already high, but when he strained to lift heavy cargo, his blood pressure went even higher, causing rupture of a small artery in his left cerebellum.

Aneurysms and Vascular Malformations

Bleeding also can ensue from abnormal blood vessels. *Aneurysms* are out-pouchings from arteries, as illustrated in Figure 3-6A. They are most often located on the large arteries that travel along the base of the brain. They are especially common at branch points where two arteries come

> Aneurysms are outpouchings from arteries.

together. The walls of aneurysms are often weak in spots. These weak spots may break, especially if the blood pressure is high. Rupture of aneurysms is usually into the subarachnoid space. Blood under arterial pressure suddenly enters the fluid around the brain, abruptly increasing the pressure within the head. If the bleeding is severe, the individual may die quickly, even before reaching a hospital. Many patients with sub-arachnoid hemorrhage report the sudden onset of the worst headache of their life. Once an aneurysm has ruptured, there is a greatly increased likelihood that it will rupture again, often soon after the first subarach-noid bleed. Occasionally, aneurysms rupture into the brain, or more often into both the subarachnoid space and the brain. Although weak places within the artery are likely to be present from birth, hypertension and other factors can lead to a gradual increase in the size of aneurysms.

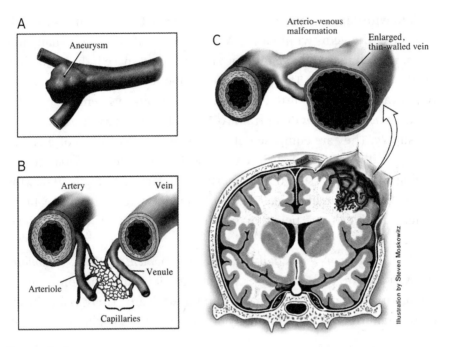

Figure 3-6

(A) An aneurysm located at the bifurcation of an artery. (B) Normal communication between an artery, capillaries, and a vein. (C) An arterio-venous malformation.

Vascular malformations, also called *angiomas,* are congenital "birth marks" that involve blood vessels. They usually arise from a failure in normal development of the vascular networks present in the fetus before birth. Some malformations are acquired during life. There are five types of vascular malformations. These types are quite different, and their names and differences are complex and confusing; they are discussed here in detail:

Arterio-venous malformations (AVMs) contain arteries that communicate directly with veins. In a normal situation, blood goes from large to small arteries (*arterioles*), and then to a bed of tiny blood vessels called *capillaries.* The blood is then drained by way of the veins, as illustrated in Figure 3-6B. In contrast to the normal situation, in an AVM, blood goes directly from arteries to veins without any intervening capillary network, as illustrated in Figure 3-6C. Veins have thin walls, and are not built to withstand the pressure present in the arterial system. As a result, rupture of the veins within an AVM is common. Bleeding is usually into the brain, but it can also be into the subarachnoid space if the AVM abuts on the brain surface. The size of the component vessels that make up AVMs varies greatly, but the largest vessels are always veins.

Cavernous angiomas differ from AVMs in that they have no direct arterial supply. They are composed of a relatively compact mass of tiny capillary blood vessels located close together in a capsule that separates the angioma from the rest of the brain. This is illustrated in Figure 3-7. Most often they appear like small lakes of blood located within the brain. When they bleed, the hemorrhage is usually contained within the capsule in the brain substance.

Venous angiomas (usually called *developmental venous anomalies* [DVAs]) are the most common type of vascular malformation found in the brain by modern brain imaging and after death. There is a deficiency of draining veins in children born with DVA, so that some of the

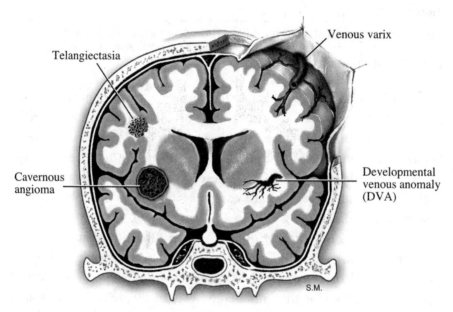

Figure 3-7

Cross section of the brain containing a cavernous angioma, developmental venous anomaly, telangiectasis, and a venous varix.

remaining veins must drain a larger portion of brain than is customary (Figure 3-7). DVAs are probably not an important cause of brain hemorrhage, but they do predispose to epileptic seizures.

Telangiectasias are tiny, dilated capillaries admixed with brain tissue and *venous varices* (extremely dilated draining veins) (Figure 3-7). They are another type of vascular malformation, but they represent very rare causes of serious brain hemorrhage.

ABNORMALITIES WITHIN THE BLOOD CAN ALSO PROMOTE BLEEDING INSIDE THE SKULL

The blood components that are effective in preventing excess thrombosis were discussed in the section under blood conditions that cause excess clotting. These same factors, when abnormal, can give rise to excess bleeding. A deficiency of blood platelets (*thrombocytopenia*) can cause hemorrhage into the skin and body organs, including the brain. A deficiency of blood clotting factors can also cause hemorrhaging. The most common such situation is the prescription of anticoagulant medications (heparin compounds, warfarin, and ximelagatran). These agents are prescribed by doctors to prevent clotting. Hemorrhage can occur when the effects of these medications are excessive. In some patients, congenital deficiency of clotting factors can lead to a lifelong risk of hemorrhage. The most well known hereditary disorder is *hemophilia*, which is a deficiency in Factor Vlll (*antihemophiliac globulin – AHG*). In patients with bleeding tendencies, hemorrhage is usually into a number of different locations, but the most devastating is bleeding into the brain.

CHAPTER 4

How Can Strokes Be Prevented? What Are the Risk Factors for Stroke and How Can They Be Reduced?

"When meditating over a disease, I never think of finding a remedy for it, but instead a means of preventing it."

Louis Pasteur

S TROKES DO NOT JUST DEVELOP "out of the blue." There are risk factors and behaviors that predispose individuals to develop a stroke. As Pasteur notes, prevention is always preferred over trying to minimize the effects

> There are risk factors and behaviors that predispose individuals to develop a stroke.

of a stroke that has already occurred. This chapter discusses these stroke risk factors and will familiarize readers with their management.

TRANSIENT ISCHEMIC ATTACKS (TIAS)

The most important event requiring immediate attention is a temporary loss of normal function of part of the brain, signaling a *transient ischemic attack* (TIA). The vascular problems that cause strokes often also cause temporary symptoms. When these spells are caused by an abnormality of the blood supply to the brain, they are referred to as TIAs or sometimes "brain attacks." The symptoms of these attacks are the same as those that occur during a stroke, except that they are temporary, often lasting only a few minutes, most often less than an hour. The most frequent symptoms are listed in Table 4-1.

A TIA signals trouble in the arteries that carry the oxygen, sugar, and other nutrients necessary for survival of brain tissue. When the lack of blood flow is brief or relatively minor, temporary loss of function develops but returns to normal when blood flow is restored. TIAs are caused by temporary blockage of an artery by a passing blood clot or temporary inadequacy of blood flow through a narrowed artery. These brief attacks indicate that something is wrong with the system and warn of the possibility of a stroke. The risk of developing a stroke is highest in the hours, days, and weeks after a TIA. Immediate medical attention is strongly recommended, because no one can predict when a stroke might occur. Finding the abnormality causing the symptoms and treating it can prevent a stroke.

Robert H. had several TIAs before his stroke. The first attack lasted 15 minutes and involved numbness and weakness of his left hand and arm. He assumed that he had leaned on his hand. Two days later, shortly after he awakened in the morning, his left face and hand became numb and tingly for about 5 minutes. That same day, he had a brief attack of decreased vision in the right eye that lasted only a minute or so. He did not understand the significance of his symptoms, and sched-

Table 4-1 Common Symptoms of TIAs

Weakness of an arm or leg—or both the arm and leg on one side of the body
Numbness of the face, arm or leg—or the face, arm, and leg on one side
Temporary loss of vision in one eye
Double vision
Loss of the ability to speak normally
Incoordination of the limbs or walking
Dizziness and loss of balance

uled a routine appointment with his family physician and an eye doctor, but he had a major stroke before he saw these doctors. Had he been evaluated quickly, carotid artery disease, the cause of his symptoms, would have been detected and treated.

When doctors recognize symptoms as TIAs, they can often diagnose the medical abnormality and give treatments that can prevent a stroke from developing. Individuals who have a TIA should seek immediate care in a medical center that has the doctors and technology available to quickly determine the cause of their particular problem. Neurologists are specially trained to diagnose and care for stroke patients. Primary and comprehensive stroke centers are available. These centers have shown that they are capable of effectively diagnosing and treating patients with cerebrovascular disease. It is important to locate the centers in your area before a problem occurs.

EARLY KNOWLEDGE OF RISK FACTORS IS THE KEY TO PREVENTION

The key words related to prevention of stroke are *individual stroke risk factors*. Chapters 2 and 3 should have made it clear to readers that strokes can be caused by many different conditions. Each individual should become aware of their own risks and behaviors that might predispose them to have a stroke. This should be done at a relatively early age. Prevention should begin early in life and continue throughout life. There is much that everyone can and should do to prevent stroke. Many of the risk factors for stroke are also risks for heart disease, so stroke prevention can also reduce the risk of a heart attack and development of heart disease.

Some risk factors are beyond individual control. For instance, we know that age, male sex, and a history of stroke in close family mem-

Some risk factors are beyond individual control.

bers are risk factors for stroke. You are more likely to have a stroke as you get older. Your chances of stroke before the age of 60 are higher if you are a man than if you are a woman. If a parent or sibling has coronary heart disease or stroke, you have a higher chance of stroke than a person whose family members do not have a history of vascular disease. But, of course, you cannot choose your parents or your sex, and living long enough to become old is a goal that everyone shares.

Unfortunately, many individuals think of risk factors and prevention only after they have had a stroke or heart attack. Prevention after an event is called *secondary prevention*, and is like shutting the barn door after the horse has already escaped, if the event is a bad stroke or a severe heart attack. *Primary prevention*, that is, prevention before a condition occurs is much preferred. We now know that most medical risk factors, and the situations that increase stroke risk, begin early in life. When teenagers and young people in their twenties die because of accidents, their blood vessels often show early indications of atherosclerosis, a degenerative condition that leads to heart attacks and strokes, and increases with time.

The author once attended a presentation by an Alabama school teacher that brought home the message that risk factors can develop early in life. This teacher asked her 6th grade students about medical conditions that had occurred in their own families. Most of the children knew very little about the medical history of their families. After all, most parents do not want to frighten their children with this type of knowledge. The teacher gave the children a homework assignment: "Go home and ask your father and mother, and any older brothers and sisters about their medical conditions, and about illnesses among grandparents and other close relatives such as aunts and uncles. Bring back this information to the class." The teacher asked a pediatrician to examine the children after their families' medical conditions had been recorded.

When the parents were shown to have a history of high blood pressure, their sons and daughters often had blood pressure that was higher than average for their age. When the family history included diabetes, the students often had higher than normal blood sugar. When mom or dad was obese, their children were often heavy. Risk factors for vascular disease are often present very early in life and should be addressed early—before the damage occurs.

Risk factors can be divided into those that are medical and those that relate to a variety of different activities, lifestyles, and behaviors. Many medical conditions, including stroke, can be prevented or minimized by medical treatments and changes in behavior.

MEDICAL RISK FACTORS

Hypertension

As discussed in Chapter 3, high blood pressure (hypertension) is the single most important risk factor for stroke. High blood pressure is very

> High blood pressure is very common.

common. Most individuals over 60 have higher than normal blood pressure. Hypertension is especially common among African-Americans and Asians, and often runs in families. Hypertension is very common in individuals who are overweight and those with diabetes.

Studies show that high blood pressure is under-recognized and undertreated. One study of 50 million Americans found that a third of patients (16 million) had high blood pressure but did not know it. Another 7.5 million individuals (15%) had hypertension but received no treatment. About a quarter of the patients (13 million) received treatment, but their blood pressures were not well controlled. Only 13.5 million (27%) individuals had hypertension that was well controlled by treatment.

Unfortunately, measurement of blood pressure at the doctor's office every few months does not give a true picture of the average level of blood pressure. Patients often become nervous when seeing a doctor, causing their blood pressure to rise. This is called "white-coat hypertension." However, these same individuals often have elevated blood pressure when confronted with stressful situations in their everyday lives. Multiple measurements of blood pressure in different circumstances and at different times of the day can give treating doctors more of a true pattern of blood pressure than infrequent measurement in the doctor's office. Blood pressure measuring devices are inexpensive and readily available. Doctors also can order a monitoring device that records blood pressure throughout the day and at night. This will provide them with the information necessary to prescribe the best treatments to keep blood pressures at normal levels. Blood pressure should be checked routinely, even in young people.

Changes in activity level and diet can reduce elevated blood pressure. Individuals who are overweight can reduce their blood pressure substantially by losing weight. Regular physical exercise, decreasing alcohol intake, and reducing salt in the diet are also useful blood pressure–reducing measures. Do not add salt to food at the table or while cooking. Check nutrition labels for the word *sodium*, including sodium chloride (table salt), sodium alginate, sodium benzoate, sodium bicarbonate (baking soda), and monosodium glutamate (MSG). Use pepper, fresh herbs, or citrus zest to add flavor to foods instead of ordinary table salt. Birth control pills can elevate blood pressure substantially in some women, and stopping this medication may return blood pressure to normal. Medicines to control hypertension have proliferated during the last decades, and treatment for each individual has to be tailored and monitored. Table 4-2 lists various classes of medications, and common medications within each class, that are prescribed by doctors to lower blood pressure.

Robert H., the first patient introduced in Chapter 1, had a family history of hypertension, and he himself had had high blood pressure for 20 years before his stroke. The stroke that he developed was due to severe carotid artery disease, undoubtedly related to his poorly controlled long-term hypertension. Tom M. had been told that his blood pressure was high, but he ignored this warning. He developed a brain hemorrhage caused by uncontrolled high blood pressure.

Diabetes

Hypertension is more common in diabetics than in individuals who have normal blood sugar.

Table 4-2 Drug Classes Used to Treat Hypertension

Diuretics
hydrochlorothiazide (Hydrodiuril®)
chlorthalidone (Hygroton®)
indapamide (Lozol®)
furosemide (Lasix®)
ethacrynic acid (Edecrin®)
spironolactone (Aldactazide®)
dyrenium (Dyazide®)
amiloride (Moduretic®)

Adrenergic nervous system agents
Beta-blockers
propanolol (Inderol®)
atenalol (Tenormin®)
Metoprolol (Lopressor®)
Nadolol (Corgard®)
Alpha-blockers
doxazosin (Cardura®)
terazosin (Hytrin®)
prazosin (Minipress®)
Combined alpha and beta blockers
labetalol (Normodyne®)
carvedilol (Coreg®)
Centrally acting adrenergic inhibitors
clonidine (Catapres®)
methyldopa (Aldomet®)
Peripherally active adrenergic inhibitors
reserpine (Serpasil®)
guanethidine (Ismelin®)

Calcium channel blockers
verapamil (Calan®)
amlodipine (Norvasc®)
nicardipine (Cardone®)
nifedipine (Procardia®)
diltiazem (Cardizem®)
felodipine (Plendil®)
Agents affecting angiotensin converting enzyme (ACE)
ACE inhibitors
perindopril (Aceon
lisinopril (Zestril®)
captopril (Capoten®)
enalapril (Vasotec®)
ramipril (Altace®)
trandolapril (Mavik®)
quinapril (Accupril®)
ACE receptor blockers
losartan (Cozaar®)
valsartan (Diovan®)
irbesartan (Avapro®)
candesartan (Atacand®)
Vasodilators
hydralazine (Apresoline®)
minoxidil (Lonitin®)

There are two well recognized forms of *diabetes mellitus*: *type 1* and *type 2*. Type 1 diabetes is due to a deficiency of insulin, the hormone secreted by the pancreas, which is responsible for the way the body uses sugar for energy. People with type 1 diabetes need to inject insulin or they will develop high blood sugar, thirst, frequent urination, and

Hypertension is more common in diabetics than in individuals who have normal blood sugar.

weight loss. Type 1 diabetes often develops in childhood or during early adult life.

Type 2 diabetes usually develops in adulthood, and is most common in overweight individuals. Unfortunately, it is now occurring often in children who are overweight. Unlike type 1 diabetics, the pancreas of these individuals produces insulin, but the insulin does not use blood sugar efficiently. Type 2 diabetes is often managed by diet and medications that help lower blood sugar. Table 4-3 lists some of the medications used to control diabetes.

Diabetes can be hereditary, and the development of diabetes in the children is almost certain when both parents have diabetes. During the last 20 years, there has been a dramatic increase in the frequency of diabetes—almost an epidemic. Some of this increase is explained by more efficient

> Diabetes can be hereditary.

diagnosis. Diabetes is especially common in individuals who are overweight, and the near epidemic may be related to the increase in the proportion of the population that is significantly overweight or frankly obese. Diabetes is more frequent among African-Americans and Asians than Caucasians.

Individuals at risk for diabetes must carefully watch their weight, and should follow a well rounded diet that is relatively low in calories, carbohydrates, and salt.

Table 4-3 Medications Used to Control Diabetes

tolbutamide (Orinase®)
chlorpropamide (Diabinese®)
glyburide (Micronase®)
glipizide (Glucatrol®)
repaglinide (Prandin®)
metformin (Glucophage®)
acarbose (Precose®)
miglitol (Glyset®)
pioglitazone (Actos®)
troglitazone (Rezulin®)
rosiglitazone (Avandia®)

Heart Disease

The heart is responsible for pumping blood into the arteries that supply the brain with blood. A variety of different cardiac conditions place individuals at risk for developing strokes, including:

Congenital heart disease. In some individuals, the heart is formed abnormally at birth. Separation of the two sides of the heart may be incomplete, and the heart valves or heart muscle may be abnormally formed. Defects in the septum, which divides the right heart chambers that pump blood into the lungs from the left heart chambers that supply blood to the rest of the body (atrial and ventricular septal defects, and patent foramen ovale), are relatively common, and can predispose to stroke. Clair H's stroke was caused by a blood clot that formed in a leg vein and then passed to her heart and through a patent foramen ovale on the way to her brain.

Heart valve disease. Heart valves can become thickened, causing narrowing of the outflow tract (called *valvular stenosis*), or can be leaky, allowing blood to pass in a reverse direction (called *valvular insufficiency*). A variety of different valve diseases predisposes to stroke, including congenital malformed valves, rheumatic fever and rheumatic heart disease, valve infections and inflammations, and degenerative thickening and scarring of valves. Some patients have had their diseased heart valves replaced by prosthetic valves, which are made either from animal tissues or synthetic materials. Clots and infections can form on prosthetic heart valves. Malfunctioning valves often lead to heart failure if not repaired or treated medically. (Chapter 3 contains additional information about heart valves.)

Coronary artery disease. Loss of blood flow to a portion of the heart causes loss of heart muscle, which is a kind of stroke that affects the heart. As discussed in Chapter 3, this is referred to as a *myocardial infarct,* or simply "heart attack." The resulting loss of effective pumping function can cause heart failure and allow clots to form in the heart that can be ejected into the circulation and reach the brain.

Abnormal heart rhythms. The heart cannot efficiently pump out blood when it contracts irregularly and rapidly. The most common abnormal rhythm, or *arrhythmia,* is called *atrial fibrillation.* This is a very common condition that increases in frequency with age. Inefficient contraction can lead to clots forming in the atria, with later ejection of these clots into the brain circulation. Medications can be prescribed in an attempt to return the heart rhythm to normal and maintain normal rhythm. Sometimes electrical stimulation (*defibrillation*) is used in an attempt to return the atrial fibrillation rhythm to normal. Studied have shown that prescription of anticoagulant medications, such as warfarin and ximelagatran, can greatly reduce the risk of stroke in individuals with atrial fibrillation.

High Cholesterol and Abnormalities of Blood Lipids

High blood cholesterol levels are an important risk factor for coronary artery disease. High cholesterol levels promote the formation of plaques in the arteries supplying the heart, limbs, and brain, Cholesterol and other lipids circulate in the blood attached to proteins: These are called lipoproteins. There are two main forms of cholesterol in the blood: *high-*

> High blood cholesterol levels are an important risk factor for coronary artery disease.

density lipoproteins (HDL), which contain the so-called "good cholesterol," and *low-density lipoproteins* (LDL), which contain the so-called "bad cholesterol." Low levels of HDL and high levels of LDL are risk factors for heart disease and stroke. An increase in *triglycerides* can also promote plaque formation and predispose to strokes. A high content of another lipid substance, *lipoprotein a* (LP a), has also been associated with an increased frequency of stroke and coronary artery disease. Lipids are derived from fats that are eaten and stored in the body.

People who have family members with high cholesterol levels are more likely to also have high cholesterol. Recognizing blood lipid abnormalities early in life can lead to effective lowering of the abnormalities by diet, exercise, and sometimes medication. It is important to know your cholesterol and other blood lipids levels. Doctors can order lipid analyses that measure the amounts of the various types of lipid substances in your blood. High blood cholesterol and other abnormalities of blood lipids can be effectively reduced by medicines (Table 4-4). Some medications have more effect on certain lipid elements than others, and sometimes doctors prescribe combinations of these medications.

Some of the medicines used to lower cholesterol, especially the class of drugs called *statins*, have additional functions that can limit the risk of strokes. Statins affect the cells lining the blood vessels (endothelium), thereby limiting the formation of atherosclerotic plaques. Even when blood cholesterol is normal, statins can reduce the buildup of plaques and may even reduce their size. Some physicians prescribe statin drugs for patients with strokes and for those with plaques who have not yet had strokes in order to reduce plaque development and enhance plaque reabsorption. Statins may also have a protective effect on the brain by increasing the brain's resistance to reductions in blood flow.

Table 4-4 Drugs Used to Reduce High Blood Lipid Levels and to Reduce Atherosclerotic Plaque Formation

Statins
    atorvastatin (Lipitor®)
    simvastatin (Zocor®)
    pravastatin (Pravachol®)
    fluvastatin (Lescol®)
    lovastatin (Mevacor®)
    rosuvastatin (Crestor®)
Resins
    cholestyramin (Questran®)
    colestipol (Colestid®)
    colesevelam (Welchol®)
Fibrates
    gemfibrozil (Lopid®)
    fenofibrate (Tricor®)
    clofibrate (Atromid-S®)
Omega-3 fatty acids (fish oil)
Niacin

Obesity

Being significantly overweight is a risk factor for a number of medical conditions that pose a risk for stroke. Overweight people are more likely to have high blood pressure, diabetes, and high blood cholesterol. These conditions often occur together. The components of this *metabolic syndrome* include obesity, high blood sugar, elevated blood cholesterol, and high blood pressure. Obesity is related to genetic factors and

> Obesity is related to genetic factors and lifestyles.

lifestyles. Clearly, overeating and inactivity predispose to weight gain. Obesity is more related to how much you eat rather than what you eat. A well-rounded diet that is relatively low in calories and salt, and regular exercise are the best antidotes to becoming or remaining overweight. People with elevated blood pressure, large waists, and blood lipid abnormalities, and who also have a family history of close relatives with heart disease or stroke, should make significant changes in their lifestyle. They should also take the medications prescribed by the doctor, in order to reduce their risk of developing diabetes, stroke, and heart disease.

Medical Illnesses

Many medical conditions can be complicated by strokes. Cancer, AIDS, serious infections, and inflammatory diseases, such as ulcerative colitis, Crohn's disease of the intestines, rheumatoid arthritis, and systemic lupus erythematosus (often called simply *lupus*) change the body's blood clotting functions, thereby increasing the chance of clots developing within the arteries that supply the brain.

Blood Conditions

Abnormalities of the cells that circulate within the blood (red blood cells, white blood cells, and platelets) and of the liquid portion of the blood can cause excessive clotting or bleeding. Too many red blood cells (*poly-*

cythemia) and a high percentage of the blood composed of red blood cells (high *hematocrit*) increase the thickness (viscosity) of the blood, cause sluggish blood flow, and predispose to excess clotting, especially when individuals become dehydrated. Many older people have low fluid intake. Severe *anemia* (very low red blood cell count and low hematocrit) is also a risk factor for stroke. *Leukemia* can also be associated with excess clotting or bleeding. Blood platelet abnormalities are a very important cause of disease. A very high platelet count (*thrombocytosis*) leads to clotting and slow blood flow within blood vessels. A very low platelet count causes spontaneous bleeding, sometimes within or around the brain.

A number of protein substances within the blood play a very important role in blood clotting. These substances protect us from excess bleeding, should a blood vessel be injured or cut. Some substances inhibit clotting (Antithrombin lll, Protein C and Protein S); other blood components (blood Factors ll, Vll, Vlll, IX, and X) stimulate clotting, when activated. A deficiency in antithrombin lll, or Proteins C or S, because of either a congenital or acquired deficiency, can cause excessive clotting. Deficiencies of blood coagulation factors often cause excess bleeding. The best known such deficiency is hemophilia, which is due to a deficiency of *antihemophilic globulin* (AHG) blood Factor lll. Two hereditary abnormalities, the presence of the *Leiden factor* (a deficiency of activated Protein C) and a *prothrombin* (Factor ll) gene mutation are recognized as important but infrequent causes of increased blood clotting.

Pregnancy, Oral Contraceptives, and Sex Hormones

During pregnancy and the period after pregnancy (the postpartum period), women have increased blood clotting potential. This increased clotting tendency is necessary to prevent bleeding from the uterus and to help maintain the placenta and the pregnancy; however, it also increases the risk that leg veins and other vessels will develop clots. The pregnant uterus compresses the veins that drain through the abdomen, increasing the tendency for leg vein clotting. The frequency of stroke can also be increased because of clotting in the veins within the head. Users of oral contraceptive drugs containing female hormones also have a slightly increased risk of stroke. The higher the dose, the more the risk. Low estrogen content birth control pills pose only a small risk. The presence of other potential risk factors, such as smoking, migraine, and hypertension, compound the risk of using oral contraceptives. It was once thought that female hormone replacement after menopause with estrogen, or estrogen and progesterone combinations, helped prevent heart disease and stroke, but recent studies suggest that these hormones are not protective and probably increase the risk of stroke and coronary artery disease. The use of male hormones to increase muscle mass and strength is also associated with an increased risk of vascular disease. The use of male hormones should be reserved for only those men whose bodies are deficient in these hormones. Women who take high doses of male hormones to change their appearance in order to look more masculine and less feminine also have a higher risk of stroke because of hormone use.

BEHAVIOR AND LIFE STYLES

Smoking

Cigarette smoking is strongly related to an increased risk of stroke and to increased narrowing and plaque formation in the arteries in the neck and head. This increased risk applies to middle-aged and older individuals, to both men and women, and especially to young people. In one

> Cigarette smoking is strongly related to an increased risk of stroke.

study of young adults (15–45 years old) in Iowa, smokers were found to be 1.6 times more likely to have a stroke than nonsmokers. Smoking was one of the most important risk factors among college students who later developed ischemic strokes. The length of time that someone has smoked, and the number of packs that they smoked, influences the development of atherosclerosis in the arteries that supply the brain and the heart. Smokers who stop smoking have less risk of stroke and heart attacks than those who continue to smoke. Smoking adds risk when other factors such as hypertension, diabetes, and the use of oral contraceptives are present.

Physical Inactivity

"Use it or lose it" is an adage that most people believe has some validity. Put a car, especially an old one, in a garage and fail to drive it for a while, and it may never be the same. Similarly, many body functions are so well coordinated that lack of use causes abilities and structures to whither with disuse. Regular exercise helps preserve weight, improve or preserve heart functions, reduce high blood pressure, and improve some blood lipid abnormalities. Physical exercise need not be rigorous to be healthy. Walking, swimming, and gardening are excellent physical activities if performed regularly.

Drugs

Illicit drugs, especially cocaine and methamphetamine ("speed"), have become a significant and frequent cause of both brain ischemia and brain hemorrhage in young and middle-aged adults. Crack cocaine is especially dangerous, because it causes sudden increases in blood pressure and a contraction of brain blood vessels. Amphetamines also raise blood pressure abruptly and cause brain hemorrhages. Heroin injected through the veins can cause brain and spinal cord strokes. Some people crush pills meant for oral use and inject them intravenously. Some of the particles contained in these drugs, such as the talc used for fillers, can reach the brain and eyes, leading to strokes and visual loss.

Prescription medications, even when given appropriately, can also become risk factors for strokes. Anticoagulant drugs, such as coumadin, heparin, and ximelagatran, can cause bleeding into the brain and other organs, especially if the intensity of anticoagulation—as usually measured in the case of coumadin by the INR (International Normalized Ratio)—is higher than desired. Aspirin and other antiplatelet medications, such as clopidogrel, ticlopidine, and to a lesser extent dipyridamole, can also cause bleeding. Some of the medications used to treat leukemia and other cancers can cause excess clotting or bleeding, and so lead to stroke.

Migraine

Migraine is one of the most misunderstood medical conditions. When people are asked about their understanding of migraine, they almost always define migraine as frequent, severe, blinding headaches. In fact, migraine can occur *without* headache, and when headaches occur, they can be slight and infrequent.

> Migraine is one of the most misunderstood medical conditions.

Migraine is a hereditary condition that most often begins early in life. It is more frequent in females than in males. During a migraine attack, arteries can narrow considerably, causing dizziness, disturbed vision, abnormal sensations, and other neurologic symptoms. Arteries can also dilate, meaning that their diameter widens, pressing on nerve endings on the outside of the arteries. This causes headache, often on one side of the head, and throbbing. Vomiting is also common. (See *Migraine and Other Headaches* by Young and Silberstein, 2004.)

During a migraine attack, vomiting and decreased fluid intake are common. Blood platelets are also activated. Dehydration and a tendency for increased clotting can lead to clots forming in already narrowed arteries, leading to the development of a stroke in the brain. These strokes are called *migrainous strokes*. Doctors often urge migraine patients to consume adequate fluids during a migraine. They also prescribe aspirin or other medications to prevent or minimize vasoconstriction, thus preventing migraine in some patients.

Physical Activities

A number of injuries to arteries arise from physical injuries. Head injuries can cause bleeding within and around the brain. Automobile and sports injuries can cause tearing of arteries within the neck and head that lead to strokes. These injuries are usually related to sudden head and neck movements that stretch the neck arteries. Neck manipulations are often performed by health care practitioners for neck pain and headache. Blood vessel tears (dissections) can develop after neck manipulation, leading to serious, sometimes fatal strokes.

Blood Test Markers

Doctors have started to place more emphasis on the results of various blood tests that can indicate a heightened risk for stroke or vascular disease (Table 4-5).

As discussed previously, high and very low hematocrit levels, and abnormally high platelet counts increase the risk of brain ischemia. Very low platelet counts increase the risk of bleeding and brain hemorrhage. Fibrinogen is a component of plaques within arteries and is a component of blood clots. High fibrinogen levels increase the risk of brain ischemia. High values of homocysteine and C-reactive protein (CRP) increase the risk of atherosclerosis in arteries that supply the

Table 4-5. Blood Tests Sometimes Used to Indicate Stroke Risk

Hematocrit
Platelet count
Homocysteine
C-reactive protein (CRP)
Antiphospholipid antibodies
Fibrinogen
Cholesterol and high- and low-density lipoproteins (HDL and LDL)
Triglycerides
Lipoprotein (a)

heart, limbs, and brain. Low levels of HDL and high levels of LDL increase the risk of atherosclerosis.

Phospholipids are present in some blood components and in blood vessels. Some individuals develop antibodies to phospholipids. Individuals with high levels of *antiphospholipid antibodies* have an increased frequency of miscarriage, stroke, leg vein clotting, and migraine.

Comments on Diet

Health is not determined only by what you eat. Nevertheless, many individuals are intensely focused on dietary intake as the way to prevent the development of disease. Research on the relationship between the intake of various food substances and disease is particularly difficult. In

> Health is not determined only by what you eat.

order to show that a given food substance either prevents or contributes to the development of a given medical condition, researchers want everything else to remain the same, including the intake of all other foods, genetics, behavior, and other diseases. The only variable should be the food substance being tested. Unfortunately, in real life there are many other variables, and they cannot always be controlled.

The American Heart Association and other medical organizations agree on the following nutritional recommendations to help prevent vascular disease:

- Do not overeat
- Limit salt intake
- Eat fruits, vegetables, and whole grains
- Include fish and fish oils in your diet
- Include the following foods in your diet, because they may help prevent stroke, heart attacks, and vascular disease: soy, grape, and tomato products, tea, walnuts, and almonds

CHAPTER 5

What Is the Appearance of the Brain and How Does It Work?

"From the brain, and from the brain only, arise our pleasures, joys, laughter and jests, as well as our sorrows, pains, griefs, and tears."

Hippocrates

KNOWLEDGE ABOUT THE BRAIN can help you understand stroke symptoms, abnormalities, and handicaps. This chapter introduces readers to brain anatomy and function. The vocabulary that doctors use to explain things to stroke patients and their families often contains anatomic and functional terms. Hopefully, this chapter will make it easier for readers to follow the explanations made by doctors and other health care professionals.

The brain is the most important organ in the human body. The brain controls movements, feelings, moods, thoughts, and perceptions, and makes it possible for us to explore the environment and interact with

> The brain is the most important organ in the human body.

others. Seeing, hearing, touching, speaking, and communicating are all brain functions. The brain is what makes our character, our abilities and failings, our intelligence, our feelings, and our personalities. The brain is intricate and complex, and it makes us what we are. This chapter describes the various parts of the brain as simply as possible, and illustrates how it appears from both the outside and inside.

THE APPEARANCE OF THE BRAIN

External Surface

Figure 5–1 shows the brain from the left side. Figure 5-2 shows the outside of the brain from the top. The largest part of the brain shown in these figures is called the *cerebrum*. The two sides of the cerebrum are called the left and right *cerebral hemispheres*. The hemispheres are separated into divisions called *lobes*. The different lobes of the cerebral hemispheres of the brain are shaded differently on Figure 5-1 to help identify them. These figures show just the surface of the cerebral hemispheres, not the deeper parts inside or the brainstem and cerebellum. These latter two structures are further back and below the cerebrum, which covers them in the same way a cap hovers over the rest of a mushroom.

The surface of the cerebral and cerebellar hemispheres of the brain is made up of folded raised strips of brain tissue called *gyri*. There are valleys or clefts called *sulci* between the gyri. A black line is drawn on Figure 5-1 along the *central sulcus*. The frontal lobe lies in front of the central sulcus; the *parietal lobe, temporal lobe,* and *occipital lobe* lie behind the central sulcus. These names are derived from common terms for the

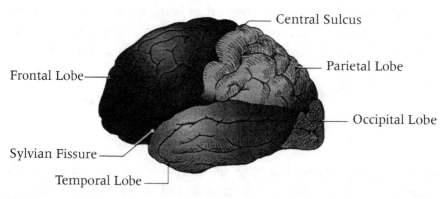

Figure 5-1

View of the cerebrum from the left side.

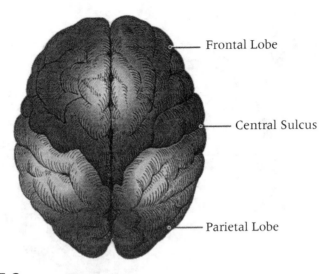

— Frontal Lobe

— Central Sulcus

— Parietal Lobe

Figure 5-2

View of the cerebral hemispheres from the top.

bony parts of the head: *frontal* comes from the front of the head behind the forehead; the temporal lobes lie behind the temples; the term *parietal* means outside or away from the center, and *occipital* comes from the Latin word that refers to the back of the head: *occi-caput*.

Figure 5-3 is a side view from the left side showing the location of the brainstem and cerebellum in relation to the left cerebral hemisphere. The brainstem is a relatively small but very critical structure located in the back of the head under the cerebrum; it connects the spinal cord below with the cerebrum above. The brainstem is an upward continuation of the spinal cord. The lowest, most *caudal* (towards the tail) portion of the brainstem is called the *medulla oblongata*. This connects to the pons, which comes from the Latin word for "bridge" because of its appearance. The most rostral (headward) portion of the brainstem is called the *midbrain* or *mesencephalon*. Above the midbrain is the *thalamus*, a region also referred to as the *diencephalon*. The brainstem has five major functions:

- It contains the nerves that relate to the head and face, and their movements and senses.

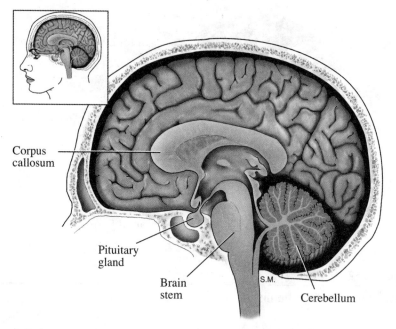

Corpus callosum

Pituitary gland

Brain stem

S.M.

Cerebellum

Figure 5-3

View of the paramedial portion of the left cerebral hemisphere and the brainstem, cerebellum, and upper spinal cord.

- It acts as a pathway for information traveling to and from the brain.
- It acts as a relay station for information coming to and from the cerebellum.
- It contains nerve cells and pathways that maintain consciousness and alertness, and relate to sleep and wakefulness.
- The nerve cells in the lower brain stem control automatic body functions, such as breathing, heart rate, and blood pressure.

Destruction of the brainstem leads to loss of all brain functions, coma, and death.

Cerebellum literally means "little cerebrum," or "little brain." It resembles a small walnut attached to the brainstem far back in the head below and behind the cerebrum, which dwarfs the cerebellum in size. The cerebellum helps coordinate all body movements, including those of the limbs, eyes, and mouth.

Internal Appearance and Composition

Figure 5-4 shows a cut section of the brain. The *cerebral cortex* is the gray ribbon on the very periphery of the section. Many of the nerve cells that relate to the various brain motor, sensory, cognitive, and behavioral functions are located in the cerebral cortex. These cortical nerve cells (called *neurons*) give rise to nerve fibers that communicate with other cerebral cortical regions. Fibers also travel from these cortical neurons downward towards the gray nuclei imbedded within the brain (often called *basal ganglia*), and also to neurons located in the brainstem, cerebellum, and spinal cord. The basal ganglia are composed of three sepa-

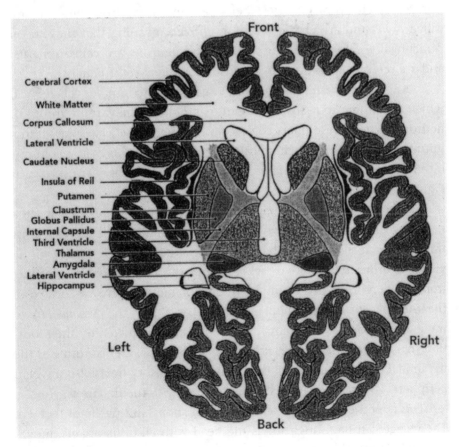

Figure 5-4

A cut section of the cerebrum.

rate but closely interrelated structures: the *caudate nucleus, globus pallidus,* and *putamen.* The caudate nucleus and putamen are often linked together as the *lentiform nucleus.*

Many fibers travel upward from the spinal cord, brainstem, cerebellum, and basal ganglia towards the cerebral cortex, primarily to relay information about the external environment and the internal environment of the body. These fibers are covered with a fatty envelope substance called *myelin,* which imparts a white color to the region under the cerebral cortex, giving rise to the term *white matter.* The myelin allows a faster transmission of nerve impulses through the nerve fibers, in the same way insulation around an ordinary electric wire facilitates the transfer of electrical energy. Fibers traveling away from neurons are called *axons* and are characterized as *efferent,* meaning that they travel centrifugally. Fibers traveling towards the neurons are called *dendrites* and are referred to as *afferent,* because they travel centripetally.

Afferent and efferent fibers are organized into bundles called *tracts,* which are similar to roads leading into and out of the various groups of neurons. When these fibers connect with other nerve cells, they transmit messages via special chemicals called *neurotransmitters* in a communication region called a *synapse.* Neurons and their fibers are shown in Figure 5-5.

The brainstem can be compared to a small village that lies outside a major urban city. Major highways going into and out of the city must travel through this village. These roads are situated on the outside of the village in order to facilitate travel. Similarly, the long motor tracts leading from the cerebrum (for example, the major motor pathways located in the internal capsule shown in Figure 5-6A), including the *pyramidal tracts,* travel in the base of the brainstem through areas named after their location (*cerebral peduncle, basis pontis, medullary pyramid*) and continue as the pyramidal tracts in the spinal cord. The main sensory tracts also travel in peripheral zones of the brainstem on their way to the thalamus.

The hypothetical village also has local shops and traffic of its own. The village can be thought of as the head with all of its organs, movements, and attached special senses. Businesses (groups of nerve cells: *nuclei*) are located mostly in the dorsal portion of the brainstem, called

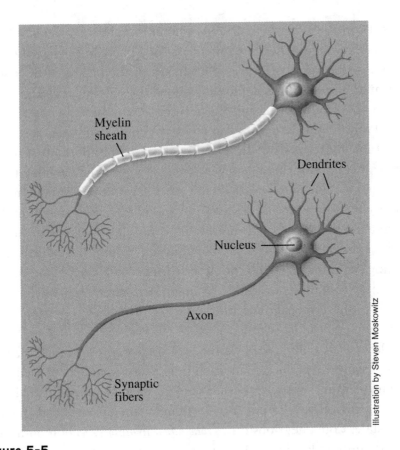

Figure 5-5

Nerve cells, axons, and myelin.

the *tegmentum*. Some of the brainstem motor nuclei control eye, tongue, face, and neck movements. Others receive sensory input related to sounds, movement in space, and touch, pain, temperature, and pressure felt in the face, throat, mouth, nose, and ears. These things all relate to local business in the village (head organs).

The cerebellum can be thought of as a separate structure that is located outside of the village. It can only be reached through the village by three different roads (the *superior, middle,* and *inferior cerebellar peduncles*), which attach to the brainstem in its lower (medulla), middle (pons), and upper (midbrain) portions. The cerebellum coordinates eye, neck, tongue, and body movements; it intimately relates to the *vestibu-*

lar system in the brainstem. The peripheral receptors for the vestibular system are located within the inner ear. They relate to a series of canals that are shaped similar to tires. Movement of the head and neck send the water in these canals in motion and tell the individual precise information about movement and the relation of the head to space. (This type of information about motion and localization in space is absolutely critical for birds and fish.) Humans get this type of information from a number of inputs, including the vestibular system, vision, and joint position sense. Information goes from the inner ears in the vestibular nerves to the vestibular nuclei located within the brainstem tegmentum. The information then goes to the nuclei that control eye movements so that your eyes move with your head, allowing you to continue to focus while running, swimming, or turning. It also goes to the cerebellum to help coordinate walking and use of the limbs. The cerebellum sends information to the cerebrum and the spinal cord nerve cells by way of the brainstem.

Alertness is maintained by a series of small neurons (called the *reticular activating system*) located on each side, near the middle of the brainstem tegmentum. These nerve cells send messages through the thalamus to each side of the cerebrum in order to maintain alertness and an energized state. Coma develops if the *reticular activating system* on both sides of the brainstem is injured. This system, along with other nuclei located in the upper brainstem, also control the sleep–wake cycle.

BRAIN FUNCTIONS

Most organs, such as the liver, lungs, and skin, are relatively homogeneous: One part of these organs looks and works the same as another. This is not the case in the brain. The structures and functions of the brain are quite well localized, and the various brain regions look and function differently. For example, moving a limb, feeling something in a hand, seeing, talking, reading, smelling, walking, hearing, and many other key bodily functions are all localized to very different but characteristic brain regions. To make things even more complex, the sides of the body, and even the functions of the individual limbs, are controlled from different localizations within the brain. The left side of the brain generally controls activities of the right arm and leg; it is involved in the perception and analysis of various stimuli (feeling, sound, and visual

> The most common disorder affecting a local region of the brain is stroke.

objects), which are presented to the right side of the body and the right side of space outside of the body. The right side of the brain controls the same functions on the left side of the body. Many psychologic and general medical problems show general symptoms of brain dysfunction, including feeling depressed, tired, sleepy, confused, and generally weak. The most common disorder affecting a local region of the brain is stroke.

MOTOR FUNCTIONS (MOVEMENT, STRENGTH, COORDINATION, AND WALKING)

In general, the parts of the brain in front of the central sulcus (the frontal lobes) are mostly related to *action* and *movement*, the so-called *motor functions*. The areas behind the central sulcus are more involved with sensory input. Figure 5-6A, B and 5-7A are diagrams of the efferent motor pathway, which originates from the primary motor cortex primarily localized to the *precentral gyrus*. The efferent pathway from the motor cortex neurons is called the *cortico-spinal* or *pyramidal tract*. This tract descends within the white matter under the cortex (called the *centrum semi-ovale*) into the white matter near the deep gray nuclei (called the *corona radiata*). The tract next courses through the front portion of the *internal capsule*, a white matter tract with a single, nearly 45-degree bend between various basal gray nuclei. This tract then descends within the basal portion of the brainstem. Fibers within the pyramidal tract will leave the main path to synapse with the various nuclei within the brainstem that control movements of the eyes, face, jaw, and tongue. The pyramidal tract then descends into the spinal cord to synapse on motor neurons within the anterior horns of the spinal cord, which innervate

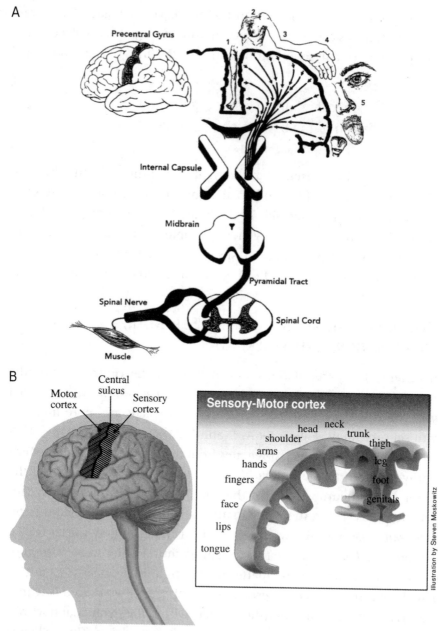

Figure 5-6

(A) The motor system. (B) The location of the motor cortex, central sulcus, and sensory-motor cortex, including detailed insert showing the parts of the body along the motor cortex.

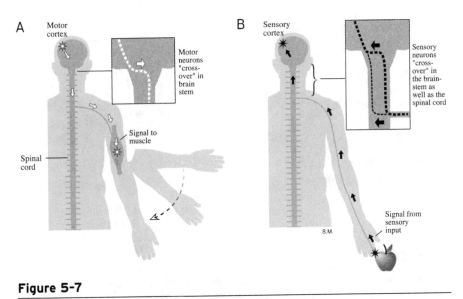

Figure 5-7

The pathways of the (A) motor and (B) sensory systems.

the muscles of the trunk and limbs. Fibers that influence voluntary movement of the upper limbs leave the tract in the upper neck (cervical portion of the spinal cord); fibers that influence the lower limbs leave the tract in the lower back (lumbar region). Some fibers within this descending motor tract go all the way to the lower end of the spinal cord (sacral or tail region) and synapse with the nerve cells that help control the pelvic and genital muscles, which relate to urination, defecation, and sexual function. Figure 5-8 shows the spinal cord and the location of the motor and sensory tracts within the spinal cord. Damage to the motor cortex or this pathway at any point leads to loss of voluntary motor control of any parts below the interruption. When the pyramidal tract or the fibers leading into it are interrupted, individuals will not be able to move their arm, hand, and leg at will. (The parts of the motor system are labeled on Figure 5-6B.)

The basal ganglia and the *substantia nigra* (a black nucleus in the midbrain) also influence motor functions. Loss of function in this area contributes to Parkinson's disease. These portions of the brain are most concerned with the automatic functions that occur without the individual thinking about them, such as the position of the body when stand-

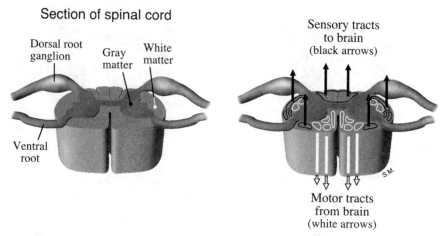

Figure 5-8

The anatomy of a cross section of the spinal cord and the general location of the motor and sensory tracts in the spinal cord.

ing and sitting, position and movement of the arms and legs while walking, and facial expression. The basal ganglia also have important functions in relation to whole body movements, such as sitting down, rising from a chair, and turning in bed.

The cerebellum coordinates and fine tunes movements and actions initiated through the basal ganglia and cortico-spinal systems. The coordination of eye movements, speech, movements of the arms and legs, and walking are influenced greatly by the cerebellum.

SENSORY FUNCTIONS

The parts of the brain behind the central sulcus (the parietal, temporal, and occipital lobes) are related to *sensory* functions: perceptions of various stimuli in the environment such as vision, sound, and touch. In contrast to the predominantly efferent (outgoing) motor system, the sensory systems convey information to the cerebral cortex so that individuals become consciously aware of what they see, hear, feel, taste, and smell. Additional input relays information about movement within space and the relation of the body to space. In general, these afferent (incoming) systems have a common general pattern. Simple stimuli are first perceived in special gyral regions. These areas are called *primary cortical regions*, and are often named by the nature of the stimulus followed by a "1." For example, primary visual cortex is called V_1, primary auditory cortex is called A_1, and touch (*somatosensory* input) is first received at S_1. The stimuli that reach these primary areas are usually very simple. For example, spots, lights, and lines are at V_1; simple sounds and noise are at A_1; and simple touches and pressures on the skin are at S_1.

Secondary sensory cortical regions, in which more elaborate sensory information is analyzed and processed, are adjacent to these primary sensory regions. In the visual sphere, these might be boxes, circles, or forms. Adjacent to the secondary cortical regions are tertiary zones that process even more complex information, such as faces, animals, and scenes in the visual sphere, and words and musical phrases in the auditory sphere.

The various cortical zones described are labeled on Figure 5-9. The visual cortical zones are mostly located in the occipital lobes; the somatosensory cortical areas are located in the parietal lobes; and the auditory regions are located in the temporal lobes. Smell and taste are also localized to the temporal lobes.

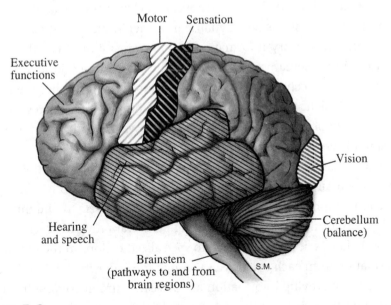

Figure 5-9

Specialized brain regions.

Sensory receptors on the periphery (within the eyes, ears, nose, tongue, and skin) first receive input from the environment. The somatosensory receptors within the skin and the bone and joints send information to the neurons within *nerve ganglia* that lie outside the spinal cord. These neurons send information about touch, pain, heat, cold, pressure, and the location of the limbs in space, toward the brain. They also send information locally to the motor nerve cells so that automatic reactions (reflexes), such as limb withdrawal, can occur without the need for the information to pass through the brain. The tracts for pain and temperature sensation (*spino-thalamic tracts*) cross to the opposite side of the spinal cord and then ascend toward a very large, centrally located structure called the *thalamus*, which sits on top of the brainstem and at the foot of the cerebral hemispheres, and serves as the main way station or relay for sensory input to the brain. Sensors specialized for motion and the position of joints and limbs send information through a different pathway. The sensory ganglia send information in a tract in the back portion of the spinal cord called the *posterior columns*. These fibers cross in the brainstem and form a tract called the *medial lemniscus*, which also travels to the sensory nuclei in the thalamus. Fibers from these two systems both synapse in nuclei in the lateral parts of the thalamus. The sensory information is then transmitted from the thalamic nuclei to a somatosensory area in the parietal lobe located in and around the post-central gyrus. When the information reaches the brain, the individual becomes aware of sensory input and changes on the opposite side of their body. (Figure 5-7B shows the pathways for transmission of sensory information.)

The visual and auditory systems relay important information to the conscious brain in a similar pattern. In each, information is first perceived in peripheral receptor nerve cells in the eye (*retina*) and inner ear (*cochlea*). Information then goes through the brain toward special nuclei in the thalamus; it is then relayed to specialized regions in the brain. The information from each eye travels through the *optic nerve* behind the eye. The fibers conveying information about visual stimuli coming from the outside parts of vision are called *temporal fields* because they are close to the temple. They travel in the inner portions of each optic nerve. The

The visual and auditory systems relay important information to the conscious brain in a similar pattern.

fibers conveying visual data about the inner portions of the visual fields are called *nasal fields* because they are close to the nose. They travel in the outer portions of each optic nerve. The inner fibers in each optic nerve then cross in an X-shaped structure near the pituitary gland called the *optic chiasm*. As you can see in Figure 5-10, this crossing realigns the

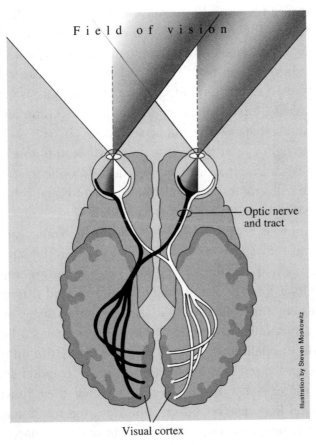

Figure 5-10

The visual pathways.

visual fibers so that visual information related to the right side of vision in each eye is now grouped in a fiber bundle that travels at the base of the left side of the brain, called the *optic tract*. This tract contains information from the right temporal visual field and the left nasal field; that is, if you drew a line directly in the middle of your vision, everything that is on the right would be contained in the left optic tract. Similarly, the right optic tract contains information from all the visual stimuli on your left (the left temporal field and right nasal field). Each optic tract synapses in a specialized visual nucleus in the back and lateral portion of the thalamus on each side, called the *lateral geniculate bodies*. In turn, fibers travel on each side within the back part of the brain in the visual radiations (called the *geniculo-calcarine tracts*) to end up in the visual cortex in the occipital lobe. The left visual cortex receives visual information from the right side of visual space, and the right visual (*striate*) cortex receives information from left visual space. The concept that the brain is organized in relation to the sides of visual space is very difficult for laypersons to grasp because they tend to think of vision solely in relation to the individual eyes. As can be seen from Figure 5–10, an abnormality in the right eye or right optic nerve will lead to loss of vision in that eye. In contrast, an abnormality in the right optic tract, right lateral geniculate body, right visual radiations, or right visual cortex will lead to vision loss in the left side of visual space.

Sound input is received by nerve cells in the inner ear, and then travels within the *auditory nerves* to nuclei located in the lateral portion of the brainstem (pons) on each side. These nuclei are appropriately named the *auditory nuclei*. Information is then relayed through a number of brainstem nuclei, finally arriving at specialized nuclei on each side of the thalamus called the *medial geniculate bodies*, which lie near but inside of the specialized visual nuclei. From here, the information is relayed to specialized hearing cortex in each temporal lobe, called *Heschl's gyri* after the individual who discovered their functions. The right temporal lobe receives information from the left side of auditory space; the left temporal lobe subserves right auditory space. Similar to the visual system, if an abnormality develops in the left ear or left auditory nerve, you will have difficulty hearing sounds exposed to the left ear. An injury to the left medial geniculate body or left temporal lobe involves all sound coming from the right side of auditory space, irrespective of which ear hears the sounds.

The thalamus also connects to regions of the cerebral cortex on each side, which have specialized abilities for memory, language, visual-spatial, and other cognitive and behavioral functions. These connections are organized as circuits in which there is reciprocal connectivity between the thalami, basal ganglia, substantia nigra, and the different regions of the cerebral cortex.

LANGUAGE AND SPEECH

Language is extremely important for daily communication. The ability to use written language, to read and write, separates humans from all other species. Speech consists of two different components: language

> The ability to use written language, to read and write, separates humans from all other species.

and the mechanical movements of the mouth lips and tongue that allow humans to articulate language. The language functions are primarily localized to a region surrounding the large fissure that separates the frontal and temporal lobes on the outer surface of the brain (the *sylvian fissure*) in the so-called dominant hemisphere of the brain. The hemisphere that is dominant for speech is nearly always the left cerebral hemisphere in right-handed individuals and in 80% of left-handers. People who are left-handed are more likely to have speech functions in each hemisphere. They will have aphasia when either hemisphere is damaged; however, the aphasia will be less severe than if speech only resided on one side. (*Aphasia* is the term used for severe loss of language capabilities.) More women have bilateral speech representation than men.

Voluntary motor control of the face and limbs on the opposite side of the body is localized to the motor strip located in the precentral gyrus. The foot of this region, just near the sylvian fissure below, is specialized for voluntary control of the muscles of the face, tongue, cheeks, and pharynx. The motor speech region, usually referred to as *Broca's area* after Paul Broca, a French physician and anthropologist, is located just below and behind this motor region. This area is located in the third frontal gyrus in a triangular region that forms a lip over the sylvian fissure (*frontal operculum*). Individuals who have injuries, infarcts, or hemorrhages in this general region, including the regions around Broca's area, often have difficulty producing normal speech. Their speech output is reduced and effortful; letters and words are poorly pronounced. The speech produced is usually accurate but not grammatically correct. Writing may also be agrammatical and telegraphic. This type of abnormality is usually referred to as *Broca's aphasia*. Most patients with this problem also have some degree of paralysis of their right hand, arm, and face.

Hearing is localized within the temporal lobes on each side. Adjacent to this region in the dominant temporal lobe is a region specialized for the understanding of spoken language. This region in the back portion of the superior temporal gyrus is usually called *Wernicke's area*, after German neurologist Carl Wernicke, who was a pioneer in the study of language and the brain. Individuals with stroke-related damage to this region use wrong and sometimes nonexistent words, and have difficulty repeating and understanding what is said to them. They may not be aware that their speech is abnormal. They may also not be able to understand what they read. Their writing also contains many wrong words. Damage limited to brain regions near Wernicke's area can cause difficulty repeating spoken language with relative preservation of understanding of speech (so-called *conduction aphasia*). Some individuals with very small lesions in the temporal lobe have a selective problem hearing words, although they can hear and identify sounds well and can speak almost normally (*pure word deafness*). Others appear as if they are deaf to language and other sound input, although they jump and blink reflexively at loud unexpected noises in their environment (*cortical deafness*).

Written language is mostly localized to a region surrounding the angular gyrus within the inferior back portion of the parietal lobe within the dominant cerebral hemisphere. Strokes and other causes of damage to this region cause individuals to become functionally illiterate. They are no longer able to read, write, and spell correctly. The inability to read and write is usually referred to as *alexia with agraphia*. Comprehension and repetition of spoken speech, and the use of wrong words depends on whether the injury also involves the temporal lobe.

MEMORY

Memory storage functions are thought to be localized into a region called the *Papez circuit,* so-named after James W. Papez, the American anatomist who first identified it. The structures within this circuit are mostly located in the medial parts of the temporal lobes on both sides and the medial portion of the thalamus and a structure called the *fornix,* a fiber band that connects the temporal lobe and the thalamus. Several key nuclear structures within the temporal lobes, called the *hippocampi* and the *amygdaloid nuclei,* play an important role in the retention of memories. The hippocampi are shaped similar to sea horses and are located adjacent to the temporal horns of the lateral ventricles of the brain. The amygdaloid nuclei are adjacent to the hippocampi and are almond-shaped. Some of the structures that play a role in memory functions are in the frontal lobes. The most important of these are the *cingulate gyri,* which are located just above the *corpus callosum* on both sides of the brain. Figure 5-11 shows the hippocampus and its location.

Memory functions can be divided into four parts: registration, reinforcement, storage, and retrieval. A person must be attentive and interested in being able to later recall certain information in order to initial-

> The ability to retain information is enhanced if a person consciously tries to retain the material.

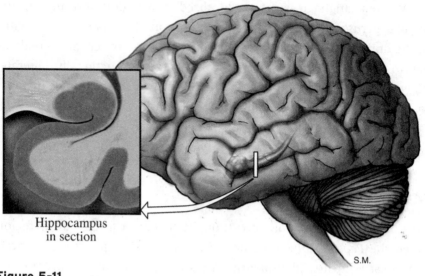

Hippocampus
in section

S.M.

Figure 5-11

The insert shows the hippocampus and its location as viewed from the outer aspect of the brain.

ly register and retain it in their brain. If you are thinking about something else or daydreaming while being told something, you will not recall it later. The ability to retain information is enhanced if a person consciously tries to retain the material. This is done by repeating the information or by associating it with something else to reinforce it. For example, a person might recall a name such as *Blaire* because it resembles their sister's name *Claire*, or because it rhymes with *fair*. Once it is reinforced and repeated, it is probably stored within structures in the Papez circuit for later retrieval.

Information is stored in the brain for later retrieval in a way similar to files in a filing cabinet. Retrieval of information is probably begun in the frontal lobes, which access the stored information in the Papez circuit. If asked to recall the name of your third grade teacher, most people will try to bring up that information by imagining themselves in their former school. They might recall the lunch their mother packed, the little girl with pigtails who sat in the row next to them, or playing with friends. They might try to visualize the teacher in front of the class. Similarly, if asked the name of a fruit, most people will try to visualize the fruit or recall its taste in order to enter their mental "fruit file." Patients with frontal lobe strokes or Alzheimer's disease often have difficulty retrieving memories and ordering them chronologically. Patients with temporal lobe lesions often have difficulty with memory storage. The left temporal lobe and thalamus are specialized for word and language memories; the right temporal lobe and thalamus are specialized for visual memories.

Memory and language are two functions that organize and integrate the sensory and perceptual functions of the brain. Having discussed these two integrative functions and some of the various forms of perception, including vision, hearing, feeling, and motor function, the following briefly discusses general patterns of cerebral hemisphere functions.

One important theme of the cerebral functions is the interrelationship between motor and sensory functions. Using vision as an example, suppose you see a picture of a scene. Most observers first *see* a key element within the scene. This is done within the *striate visual cortex* within the *occipital lobes*. This initial visual information generates questions that the viewer tries to answer by looking further at the picture. Eye movement searches are generated by the frontal lobe gaze centers. This looking induces further input of visual information, which, in turn, raises further questions and stimulates more looking. Gradually, the viewer gets more and more information from the picture. This process of exploration, a motor behavior called "looking" in the visual sphere, and a perceptual activity referred to as "seeing" in the visual sphere together result in acquiring maximum information.

The information acquired by an individual depends on their level of interest, intelligence, and experience. Referring to the memory zones within the temporal lobes and thalami and the language area in the left

> The information acquired by an individual depends on their intelligence and experience.

perisylvian areas supports the interpretation of visual information and the ability to name the various things seen. Similarly, if you are blindfolded and something is placed in your hand, you will feel it and generate possibilities regarding the nature of the object. You will touch and explore the object in order to discover its nature and its name. This tactile perception takes place in the somatosensory area within the postcentral gyrus of the parietal lobe opposite to the hand in which the object was placed. The manual movements of exploration are generated in the hand and arm area of the precentral gyrus in the opposite frontal lobe. Similarly, hearing a tune being played on a piano occurs in the lateral portion of the temporal lobes. An individual will try to listen or "tune into" certain aspects of the music. This tuning is probably a frontal lobe function. Of course, as in seeing, accurate identification of the nature of the object to be felt or the music being played depends heavily on the previous experience of the individual. If they have never heard the tune or felt the object, they will not be able to identify it correctly.

Another important theme is the circuitry between perceptual regions (located behind the central sulcus) and language and memory regions. For example, suppose someone shows you a familiar coffee mug. You first *see* the cup with your eyes and your visual cortex. Transmission of the visual data to your language area in the left cerebral hemisphere will probably result in generation of the word name *mug* or *cup*. Transmission of the information to your visual memory area in the right medial temporal lobes and then the left medial temporal lobe enables you to *remember* that this particular cup was given to you as a present by your office staff and that you use the mug for coffee each morning at work. Activation of your taste regions in the temporal lobes reinforces that coffee is the only substance placed in this mug. The tactile zones in your parietal lobes might result in your recalling the feeling of the mug in your hands in the morning and that the mug is made of clay. Relay of information between the various sensory areas, the motor exploration areas, memory, and language have let you characterize the nature of that particular object.

There is also an *affective* element of perception. Some of the things that we see, hear, feel, and otherwise experience have an emotional effect upon us. These perceptions make us feel fearful, uneasy, happy, angry, excited, or sad. At times, we are quite aware of the emotional content of the perceptions, but at other times we are not. Perceptions also have a circuitry through the limbic lobes of the brain, including the temporal lobes and the cingulate gyri, that give our observations and experiences an emotional and affective value. The right cerebral hemisphere may have more influence on the emotive, affective content than the left cerebral hemisphere.

EMOTIONS, AFFECT, AND SELF-IMAGE

Strokes cause psychologic and physiologic changes in self-image. Strokes often create deficits that are easily visible to everyone, even during casual encounters with stroke survivors. Abnormalities of facial appearance,

> Strokes cause psychologic and physiologic changes in self-image.

use of the limbs, walking, and speech are often quite obvious to all observers. Patients worry whether or not the changes will prove acceptable and tolerable to others. This is especially problematic when caregivers need to significantly alter their own activities in order to help the person affected by stroke. Patients wonder whether family members will be willing and able to handle the added responsibility. Will caregivers participate with enthusiasm, or will the patient feel like an unwanted burden? Significant others must understand these worries, and try to calm and reassure patients whenever possible.

Physiologic changes due to stroke are usually in the other direction; that is, patients often do not fully comprehend the nature and severity of their deficits and are inappropriately unconcerned. The right cerebral hemisphere is important in regard to both awareness of deficits and emotive responses towards them. Some individuals with large right cerebral hemisphere strokes, who have left limb paralysis and loss of attention to their left visual field, may completely deny that anything is wrong with them. This lack of awareness of the deficit is called *anosognosia*. The author was once called to the emergency room of the hospital at 3:00 A.M. by a perplexed, desperate husband and doctor-in-training. A woman had very suddenly developed complete paralysis of her left limbs, and was brought to the hospital by her husband despite her resistance. She absolutely refused to be admitted to the hospital, declaring that nothing was the matter with her. Neither the husband nor any of the emergency room personnel had been able to convince her otherwise. Indeed, she had complete left-sided paralysis, loss of sensation in her left limbs and body, and a lack of response to objects on her left side. After the examination, she said, "You see, nothing is wrong with me." Rather than argue, she was given her car keys and told that if she could walk to her car and drive home that she could go. She tried to get up and slipped to the floor, unable to rise. She accused hospital staff of tripping her, but said that she now needed to stay because of the fall. Not until the second week of hospitalization did she develop any realization that there was something wrong with her limbs, feeling, and vision.

Emotive reactions are often blunted in patients with right cerebral damage. They often have difficulty expressing emotions in their facial expressions and voices, and may have difficulty picking up the "body language" and emotional tones of others. This abnormality of affect has been referred to as *dysprosody*, which literally means an "abnormality of the rhythm and tone of speech." Speech has two major aspects. One is *linguistic* and relates strictly to the meaning of the words used. The other aspect is *affective*. The same words can take on very different meanings, depending on tone, volume, accent, facial expression, gestures, and emphasis. The phrase "come home early," when spoken by a spouse, may have many meanings depending on how and when the words are spoken. They could mean, "If you get a chance it would be nice if you were early." They could mean "You had better be home early." The words could have a sexual or other connotation indicating some reward for an early appearance or punishment for not arriving early. The ability to transmit and interpret body language and emotional tone is an integral part of communication between individuals. Strokes, especially those in the right cerebral hemisphere, can blunt affective responses and alter nonlinguistic communications. These problems should be explained to caregivers and significant others.

CHAPTER 6

What Are the Arteries and Veins that Supply the Brain?

"All the veins and arteries proceed from the heart, and the farther away they are from the heart the thinner they become and they are divided into more minute ramifications."

Leonardo da Vinci

JUST AS A PLUMBER NEEDS TO KNOW what pipes connect to a malfunctioning sink and how those pipes carry water from the water source to the sink, doctors must try to identify the blood vessels that are blocked or leaking. Identifying the location and nature of the problem in the heart and blood vessels is important in order to choose the appropriate treatment.

Figure 6-1 shows the neck arteries that branch out from the aorta. The two main arteries are called the *carotid arteries*; they are located on each side of the front of the neck. The *common carotid arteries* are branches that arise low in the neck. On the right side, the *innominate artery* is the first large branch to come from the aorta. The innominate artery branches into the right *subclavian artery* (literally, the artery that goes under the clavicle) to supply the right arm and the right common carotid artery, which ascends on the right side of the neck. The left common carotid artery is the second major branch coming from the aorta. It ascends towards the head on the left side of the neck. The third branch from the aorta is the left subclavian artery, which supplies the left arm with blood.

Each common carotid artery branches in the neck into an *external* carotid artery and an *internal* carotid artery. The external carotid arteries

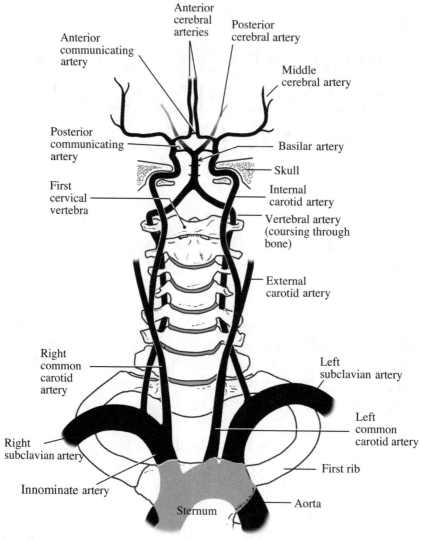

Figure 6-1

Arteries located in the neck.

supply the face and the structures within the head other than the brain, while the internal carotid arteries supply the brain and the eyes with blood. The internal carotid arteries each supply the front part of the cerebral hemisphere and the eye on the same side as the artery. The right carotid artery branches to the right eye; to the right frontal, parietal, and temporal lobes; and to the basal ganglia and internal capsule and anterior portions of the white matter in the cerebral hemispheres. The left internal carotid artery supplies the identical structures on the left side of the brain.

Inside the skull, each internal carotid artery divides into a *middle cerebral artery*, which supplies mostly the structures on the outer lateral surface of the cerebral hemispheres, and an *anterior cerebral artery*, which supplies the brain structures near the midline. Figure 6-2 shows the left carotid and left vertebral arteries, and their branches, as viewed from the left side. Figure 6-3 is a view from the bottom of the brain showing the branching of the vertebral and basilar arteries inside the skull.

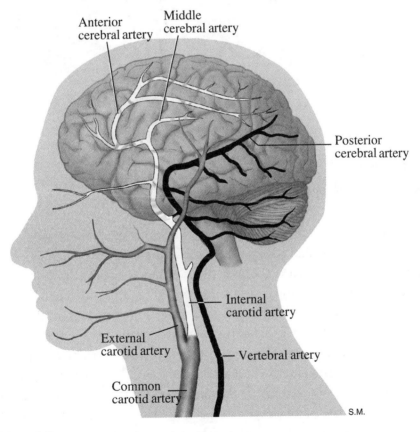

Figure 6-2

Arteries of the neck and head viewed from the left side.

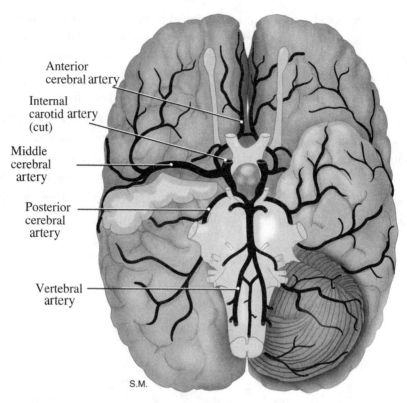

Anterior
cerebral artery

Internal
carotid artery
(cut)

Middle
cerebral
artery

Posterior
cerebral
artery

Vertebral
artery

S.M.

Figure 6-3

Vertebral and basilar artery branching within the skull.

The two *vertebral arteries* that ascend towards the brain in the back of the neck on each side nourish the parts of the brain not supplied by the internal carotid arteries. The paired *vertebral arteries* branch off from the arteries to the arms (the subclavian arteries), and pass through holes in the vertebral bodies. They eventually enter into the back of the brain through a large hole located at the point where the neck vertebrae meet the skull (the *foramen magnum*). The two vertebral arteries supply the medulla oblongata and the back undersurface of the cerebellum on each side, and then join to form the *basilar artery*, a midline blood vessel that supplies the brainstem above the medulla oblongata on both sides. The basilar artery gives off branches near its termination that supply the upper surface of the cerebellum on both sides. The basilar artery divides at a midbrain level and gives branches to the thalami and the temporal and occipital lobes of the cerebral hemispheres on each side. The end large artery branches of the basilar artery are called the *posterior cerebral arteries*. Figure 6-3 shows the supply of the vertebral and basilar arteries to the brain.

Veins are located deep within the brain and on its surface. These veins drain into large venous structures, the *dural sinuses*, located within layers of the dura mater. Blood drains into large neck veins from the sinuses, and from there into the heart. The largest neck veins are called the *jugular veins*. Fluid cannot easily drain from the head when veins become blocked, causing blood and water to build up within the brain region that is normally drained by the blocked vein.

> Fluid cannot easily drain from the head when veins become blocked.

Understanding the structure and functions of the brain, and the arterial and venous supply of the brain, will prepare readers to better understand the symptoms that can develop when an artery becomes blocked.

CHAPTER 7

What Are the Different Symptoms of Stroke? What Abnormalities Do Doctors Look for and Find in Stroke Patients?

"Listen. Listen to your patient. He is giving you the diagnosis."

Dr. Rene Laennec

"History and the physical examination provide the essential basic facts for diagnosis."

Dr. A. M. Harvey

GOOD MEDICAL CARE INVOLVES full interaction and cooperation between patients and doctors. Of course, doctors cannot treat someone unless the person comes to the doctor with their symptoms. Symptoms develop when people become aware of changes in any of the usual func-

The timing of treatment is critical.

tions of their bodies. The timing of treatment of stroke patients is critical because brain tissue is quite vulnerable to changes in blood supply. The adage *time=brain* emphasizes the importance of rapid treatment of any circulatory problem that threatens to injure the brain. You will be able to get to the doctor in time to prevent serious damage if you are aware of the symptoms that might indicate stroke.

There are two different types of symptoms—those that reflect loss of function of parts of the brain, and those that relate to the vascular cause of brain injury. The following illustrates the two types of symptoms:

Sam J., who was introduced in Chapter 1, noticed that his heart would occasionally beat fast and irregularly. This worried him, and he made an appointment with his doctor. But before he saw the doctor, one afternoon he suddenly realized that his right hand and leg had become weak. He felt tingling in the entire right side of his body, including his face. When he was examined at the hospital, the doctors noted that he had atrial fibrillation. A clot had formed in his large and inefficiently contracting left heart atrium and embolized to a blood vessel supplying the left side of the brain, causing brain infarction.

Sam's bouts of rapid irregular heartbeat were symptoms of atrial fibrillation. His right limb weakness and the numbness of his right body developed because of loss of function of an area within the left cerebral hemisphere of the brain. In very simple terms, the symptoms caused by atrial fibrillation gave a clue as to what was wrong. The nature of the brain symptoms provided information about where the problem was located in his brain.

Both the *what* and *where* questions are important. The question as to where the problem is located is similar to the plumber asking which sink or bathtub in the house is not functioning well. If there is a malfunctioning sink in the bathroom on the second floor, the plumber knows or can find the pipes that lead to that sink. He is then in a position to explore all the structures that influence those pipes and discover what is blocking the flow of water. Similarly, knowing that Sam's brain problem was located within brain tissue supplied by the left middle cerebral artery allowed the neurologist to explore that particular pathway. Clearly identifying the *what* aspect (in Sam's case, atrial fibrillation) allowed the physician to emphasize heart evaluation.

This chapter discusses the symptoms caused by abnormal brain function (the *where* question), and the symptoms that relate to the medical condition that caused the stroke (the *what* question). Readers be warned: Neither the brain symptoms nor the medical condition symptoms are specific for stroke. Loss of brain functions can be caused by many different conditions, not only stroke. Neurologic symptoms can also originate in parts of the nervous system other than the brain. Everyone has had the experience of having their hand or leg become numb when the nerves in that limb have been compressed, such as when sitting with the legs crossed for some time.

The timing of symptoms is often very important in diagnosing stroke, because strokes usually come on suddenly. A person who has a stroke is literally abruptly *stricken* with brain symptoms. Only a very small minority of strokes develop gradually.

Similarly, symptoms that accompany other, nonstroke, medical conditions can also be nonspecific, including headache, vomiting, neck discomfort, and chest pain.

SYMPTOMS DUE TO LOSS OF BRAIN FUNCTION

The following are some of the symptoms that might develop when parts of the brain stop functioning normally (refer back to Chapter 5 to clarify the brain structures involved).

Weakness

Loss of strength and coordination in one or more limbs is a common symptom of stroke. Most people equate stroke with paralysis, but although weakness is a very common symptom, many stroke patients

> Loss of strength and coordination in one or more limbs is a common symptom of stroke.

have no paralysis. The weakness can involve one body part, such as a hand, but usually it involves more than one area on the same side of the body. Sam J. noticed sudden weakness of his hand and leg. Common locations for weakness to develop in stroke patients include these combinations:

- Face, arm, and hand
- Arm and leg
- Face, arm, and leg

Occasionally, when a critical blood vessel that supplies the brainstem is involved, both sides of the body and all four limbs can become weak at the same time.

Numbness

Different people use the word "numb" to mean quite different things. The most common usage is loss of the ability to feel in the numb areas. Some people describe a loss of sensation, as if the area had been injected with novacaine. Prickling, tingling, and "falling asleep" are other descriptions that are often used. Occasionally, the sensations described are unpleasant, such as burning, hot, oversensitive to touch, or an unpleasant feeling when warm or cold objects are placed on the numb area. The numbness can involve just one limb or part of a limb, or it can involve multiple regions on one side of the body. Sometimes the numbness involves the face, arm, leg, and trunk on one side of the body. Some patients describe the feeling as if a line was drawn right down the midline of their body with everything on one side of the line becoming numb, as in Sam's case. Often numbness and weakness are described together in the limbs or face on one side of the body.

Loss of Vision

Visual loss is another common symptom of strokes and TIAs. The visual loss can involve only one eye. The first branch of the internal carotid artery is the *ophthalmic artery*, the main blood supply of the eye. Patients

Visual loss is another common symptom of strokes and TIAs.

often develop temporary visual loss in an eye when the carotid artery is narrowed. They describe it as a shade coming down from the top that gradually blocks vision in the eye. At times, the shade comes across the eye similar to a curtain being pulled from the side. Sometimes, the vision in one eye becomes grey or black. Visual loss can occur at the same time in both eyes when blood pressure becomes very low.

Interruption of blood supply often involves one or both *posterior* cerebral arteries. These are the vessels supplying the brain regions on each side of the brain that receive visual messages from objects on the opposite side of the environment. Blockage of the right posterior cerebral artery impairs vision to the left. Alternatively, vision will be impaired to the right if the left posterior cerebral artery is blocked. Some patients do not recognize the loss of their span of vision, and only become aware that something is wrong when they run into objects or cars on their blind side. At times, patients become aware of "holes" in their vision on one side. Rarely, an embolus that blocks both posterior cerebral arteries will cause patients to become effectively blind.

Dizziness, Vertigo, and Loss of Balance and Coordination

Structures in the human brainstem and cerebellum help us maintain our balance and equilibrium. Impairment of these structures results in dizziness, and sometimes severe *vertigo* occurs, the sensation that the person or the room is moving or turning. Double vision and the sensation that objects are oscillating can also occur.

This type of abnormality can involve mostly balance and walking. Individuals may veer or lean to one side, or stagger from one side to another. At times, just the limbs on one side become uncoordinated or shake (tremor) when the individual attempts to grab an object with their hand.

Speech and Language

Two different types of speech abnormalities can be symptoms of stroke: dysarthria and aphasia. Some stroke patients have difficulty pronouncing words. This abnormality, referred to as *dysarthria*, is related to weakness of the muscles that are used in talking: the face, mouth, lips, tongue, pharynx, and jaw muscles. Dysarthric patients may be difficult to understand because they slur words, but the words that they do speak are correct, and they understand speech. They can write normally if their hand is not too weak.

> Some stroke patients have difficulty pronouncing words.

As discussed in Chapter 5, aphasia (in contrast to dysarthria) is an abnormality of language. Stroke patients may use the wrong words, and the phrases that they speak may not represent correct English statements or grammar. They may be completely unable to speak. Some aphasics also have difficulty understanding the language of others, either spoken or written. These language abnormalities may include reading, writing, and spelling. Language abnormalities in nearly all right-handed, and four-fifths of left-handed individuals, are caused by strokes in the left cerebral hemisphere areas devoted to language.

Abnormalities of Memory, Thinking, and Behavior

A large part of the human brain is concerned with thinking, memory, interpreting visual space, and governing how people act. Abnormalities of these functions are common in stroke patients, but they are most often accompanied by abnormalities already discussed: weakness, numbness, visual loss, abnormal walking and coordination, and abnormal speech.

Some stroke patients develop difficulty remembering events and conversations. The *memory loss* in these patients develops suddenly. They tend to repeat stories and questions, and do not recall answers or recent events.

Some stroke patients seem to be unaware of objects or people located on one side of their physical environment. They often ignore everything and everyone on their left side. This abnormality is referred to as "neglect of one side of space." Some stroke patients lose their sense of space and proportions. They cannot recall where things are located, and cannot draw or even copy simple visual objects. They may get lost in areas that were formerly familiar to them; they may even get lost in their own house. These *visual-spatial abnormalities* are often present in patients who have stroke damage in the right cerebral hemisphere.

In some patients, the change in function relates to the quantity of their behavior and interactions. They may do much less and be content with little spontaneous action or speech. They lose interest in activities, reading, hobbies, and other people. Their families and friends may comment on their lethargy and call them "couch potatoes." Some patients may become restless and hyperactive. They may talk incessantly, much more than usual. One topic may merge into another. These individuals appear agitated, restless, and hyperactive.

USING SYMPTOMS TO DETERMINE THE LOCATION OF BRAIN DYSFUNCTION

Doctors consider all of a patient's symptoms when trying to discover where in the brain the dysfunction lies. Sam J. had symptoms of weakness in his right hand and leg, and loss of sensation involving the right limbs and right side of his body. Given these symptoms, the abnormality would have to involve the left precentral motor cortex and the adjacent postcentral gyrus sensory regions toward the top of the brain. The most lateral regions were likely spared, because his face was not affected, and he had no speech abnormalities. Sam's neurologists would have checked the motor and sensory function of his face and all aspects of his speech to be certain of his diagnosis. The general principal that neurologists use is to listen to the patient's symptoms, develop an initial impression of the probable general location in the brain, and then use this information to decide what to look for in an examination.

Robert H. suddenly developed left limb paralysis associated with neglect of the left side of visual space; he was completely unaware of his loss of function. These symptoms indicate a large abnormality in the right cerebral hemisphere. Claire's inability to speak and right limb paralysis pointed to a left cerebral problem involving the speech region on the lateral side. Tom's loss of balance in walking, lurching to the left, and dizziness suggested an abnormality in the left side of the cerebellum.

SYMPTOMS THAT RELATE TO THE CAUSE OF STROKE

There are few symptoms that are specific for stroke or for the subtype of stroke. Sam's irregular heartbeat suggested strongly that his stroke was due to embolism. In some patients, headache precedes or accompanies

> There are few symptoms that are specific for stroke.

the stroke. Headache can result from blockage of some blood vessels and dilation of other blood vessels to take up the slack. Headache can also result from high blood pressure and from bleeding into or around the brain. Tom M. had headache, vomiting, and decreased consciousness at the onset of his stroke, indicating a hypertensive brain hemorrhage.

SYMPTOMS DOCTORS LOOK FOR WHEN THEY SUSPECT A STROKE

Physical findings and symptoms are divided into those that relate to brain dysfunction and those that relate to the vascular cause. Heart and vascular examinations seek abnormalities that might be stroke-related. Doctors check the pulse at the wrist to determine the heart rate and regularity. They also check blood pressure and listen to the heart. They listen for *murmurs*, which might suggest abnormalities of the heart valves and heart contractions. They listen for *bruits*, a French term for noise that is audible along the arteries, suggesting that the artery might be narrowed at the point the bruit is heard. They may check the carotid, subclavian, and innominate artery pulses in the neck. They may also listen to the neck arteries and the eyes. Doctors may examine the abdomen and feel the pulses in the feet.

Neurologic testing varies with the type of symptoms and the time available for the examination. Neurologists look for abnormalities of brain function when examining a patient. The following is a description of a typical examination, but keep in mind that not every doctor will perform a complete examination on every patient. This example is included to familiarize patients with what the doctor may do to determine if there are abnormalities in the function of any part of the patient's nervous system.

The conversation in which the patient describes symptoms and events, and responds to questions tells the doctor about their speech, pronunciation, and their ability to understand spoken language. The doctor will often ask the patient to repeat phrases and name objects in the room to test speech further. A patient may be asked to read a paragraph in a magazine or newspaper, and to write a brief paragraph about the city where they live or another familiar topic. The doctor may show several pictures to the patient and ask her to describe the pictures after the pictures have been removed from view. This tells the doctor something about the patient's *visual-spatial* abilities. To test these functions further, the doctor may ask the patient to draw a clock, bicycle, daisy, or another familiar object from memory, and then to copy a complex diagram provided by the doctor. The patient may be asked to describe and name famous people depicted in photographs. Memory may be tested by asking the patient to try to recall the paragraph that they read, the scenes that he saw, and the individual photographs that were shown to him.

The functions of the structures in the face and head will be tested. Visual acuity in each eye will be tested with a handheld eye chart. The patient may be asked to face the doctor, who will bring a finger or an object into the patient's field of vision from each side in order to determine if peripheral vision is preserved. The doctor will use an ophthalmoscope to look at the blood vessels and the nerve within the eye. The pupil of the eye and the eyelids will be observed, and the movements of each eye and of the eyes moving together to each side and up and down will also be tested. Movements of the face, throat, and tongue, and hearing in each ear will be assessed. Feeling on the face will be tested with cotton, touch, and a cold object.

The doctor will check to see if the patient's arms are of equal strength by asking the patient to hold her arms out in front of herself so the doctor can observe if one side drifts downward, indicating weakness. The muscles of the arms at the shoulders, elbow, wrist, and hand on both sides will be tested in turn. The reflexes at the elbows and wrists will be tested with a reflex hammer. Feeling in the arms is tested using cotton, touch, and sometimes a pin. The doctor may move the fingers slightly up or down while the patient's eyes are closed in order to see if the patient can detect the movement and its direction. The doctor will also check to see if the patient can feel the vibrations of a tuning fork placed on her fingers.

The lower limbs will be tested in the same way as the upper limbs; strength, reflexes, and feeling will be analyzed. Watching the patient stand and walk is another very important part of the examination. Gait is observed as the person proceeds into the examination room, or at the very end of the examination if the doctor first met and examined the patient in a hospital bed.

Sam J. occasionally used wrong words when he was examined, and had difficulty understanding a paragraph that he tried to read. His right hand was weak, but his leg had normal strength. He was able to feel touch, cold, and the vibrations of a tuning fork normally on his right and left hands, feet, and body. These findings made it clear that his problem could only be localized to the left cerebral hemisphere, in an area near the lateral surface within and near the speech zone. Some of his symptoms had improved, and he was functioning better than he had been when he first developed neurologic symptoms.

Examination of Robert H. showed complete paralysis of his left arm, hand, and leg. He could not appreciate or localize touch or cold placed on his left side. He could not see to his left. He did not think anything was wrong with him, despite these abnormalities. He clearly had sustained severe damage to a large area on the right side of his brain.

By the time that Claire H. was examined, her speech was almost back to normal. She had some slight difficulty in repeating phrases and in understanding complex questions. The strength in her limbs was normal. The reflexes were slightly greater in her right arm and leg, compared with the left. She also had a condition that affected the lateral part of her brain on the left side.

Tom M. leaned to the left when he attempted to sit or stand. He could not walk. He lurched in a drunken fashion to his left side when he attempted to walk. His left arm and hand were quite clumsy when attempting to reach for an object. These findings reinforced the idea that his left cerebellum was not functioning normally.

Having determined the nature of the patient's symptoms and the abnormalities found on examination, the doctor is in a position to order images and laboratory tests to better pinpoint any abnormalities in the brain and in the blood, heart, and blood vessels that supply the brain.

CHAPTER 8

How Can Doctors Tell
What Caused a Stroke?
What Tests Are Used to
Evaluate Individuals Who
May Have Had a Stroke?

"For when the cause of the complaint is unsure
'Twould be a miracle to find a cure."

Miguel de Cervantes

DOCTORS ORDER LABORATORY TESTS to evaluate patients based on the nature of the symptoms and signs in each individual patient and on their stroke risk factors. This chapter describes the types of tests commonly ordered and the purposes of each test. Each patient suspected of stroke may not have all of these tests, however. The purpose of this chapter is simply to familiarize readers with testing.

Doctors are able to find out, safely and quickly, whether a person has had a stroke, and whether the stroke is due to brain hemorrhage or brain ischemia. They can determine where and how much the brain has

> Doctors are able to find out, safely and quickly, whether a person has had a stroke.

been damaged, and the presence, nature, and severity of any abnormalities affecting the blood vessels that supply the brain. Testing also shows if heart or blood abnormalities were the cause or contributed to causing the stroke. Knowing exactly what is wrong with a stroke patient allows selection of the best treatment. Stroke patients and their families should become familiar with the available tests so that they can understand what has or has not been done to investigate the stroke and the condition of the stroke patient's blood vessels.

Very important clues as to *where* the stroke is located in the brain and *what* caused it come from the history that the doctor takes from the patient and the results of the physical and neurologic examinations. Because of publicity about new technologies, many patients think that the history-taking and physical examination have been entirely replaced by tests, but this is certainly not true. Examining patients is the only way to know what they can and cannot do.

MAKING IMAGES OF THE BRAIN

There are two general types of brain imaging tests: *computed tomography* (CT) and *magnetic resonance imaging* (MRI). CT uses ordinary X-rays and computers to make images of thin slices through different levels of the brain. Each slice contains a picture of the brain structures present at that level. MRI uses magnetic energy to create images of the brain. Both tests are safe and painless. Each requires the patient to place their head into a machine, and with MRI, much of the body may also be enclosed. Patients must remain completely immobile so the machines are able to make clear, high-quality images. People who are claustrophobic may have difficulty holding still while they are in the machine. The MRI machine is also noisy.

MRI produces images of different sections of the brain and generates them at different angles. Cuts are taken from the top to the bottom (coronal), along the long axis of the brain (axial), and from side to side (sagittal). Doctors sometimes order an intravenous injection of a substance that adds contrast to the images in order to obtain more detail on the brain image. In CT this is usually an iodine-containing substance. Gadolinium is the chemical used for contrast enhancement during MRI. Occasionally, patients have an allergic response to these contrast substances, especially to the dye used for CT contrast.

CT and MRI allow doctors to separate brain hemorrhages from infarctions. They can also show whether bleeding has occurred within the skull, but outside of the brain in the subarachnoid, subdural, or epidural spaces (see the discussion and figures in Chapter 2). Hemorrhages appear white on CT scans. Infarcts are gray or black, making it quite easy to separate the two main stroke categories. Figure 8-1 is a CT scan from Robert H. showing a large brain infarct involving the right cerebral hemisphere. The small black arrows point to the infarct, which appears darker than the surrounding brain tissue. Figure 8-2 is an MRI scan of Claire H. showing a small brain infarct within the left cerebral hemisphere. The infarct appears much whiter than the surrounding normal brain. In contrast, the CT from Tom M. (Figure 8-3) shows a

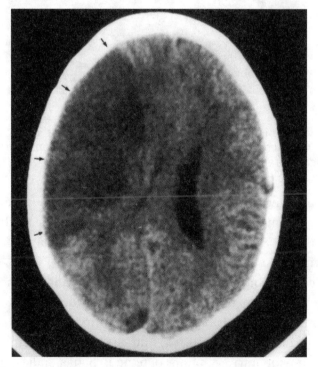

Figure 8-1

CT scan of Robert H., showing a large, right cerebral infarct. The infarct is on the left of the figure, which represents the right side of the brain. The small black arrows point to the brain infarct, which appears darker than the surrounding tissue.

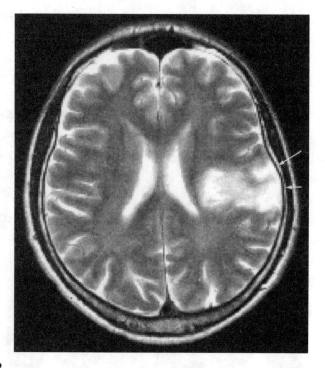

Figure 8-2

MRI scan of Claire H., showing a left cerebral infarct. The infarct appears as a white, nearly rectangular area (small white arrows) on the right of the figure, which represents the left side of the brain.

cerebellar brain hemorrhage. The region of bleeding appears more white than the surrounding tissue. The white arrow points to the area of bleeding. Figure 8-4 includes CT scans and MRI images from other patients with brain hemorrhages and infarcts.

Brain images not only show whether the lesion is a hemorrhage or infarct, they also show where the abnormality is located, how extensive it is, and whether there is brain swelling and pressure build-up caused by the infarct or hemorrhage. CT and MRI can be normal in some patients with temporary symptoms of brain ischemia, indicating that the brain has not been irreversibly damaged—that is, not yet infarcted. Knowing where the abnormality is located in the brain allows doctors to determine which blood vessels supply the abnormal region. These vessels can then be checked for abnormalities.

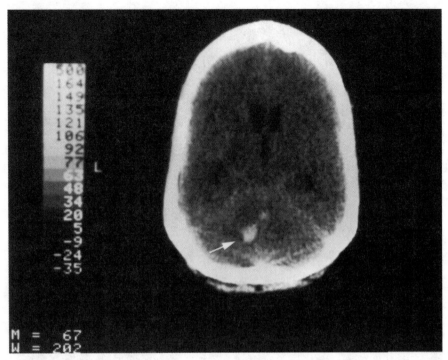

Figure 8-3

CT scan of Tom M. showing a left cerebellar hemorrhage. The hemorrhage appears white (white arrow points to the hemorrhage).

MAKING IMAGES OF THE BLOOD VESSELS AND DETERMINING BLOOD FLOW

After identifying stroke-related abnormalities in the brain, doctors test the arteries that supply the injured brain. Pictures of the arteries (*angiograms*) can be created using a CT scanner. *CT angiograms* (CTAs) are made by injecting an iodine-containing dye into an arm vein and then taking pictures rapidly as the dye goes through the arteries and veins in

> After identifying stroke-related abnormalities in the brain, doctors test the arteries that supply the injured brain.

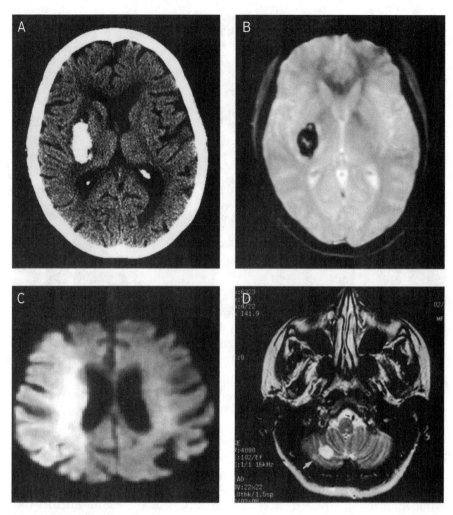

Figure 8-4

(A) CT scan showing a hemorrhage in the deep portion of the brain. The hemorrhage appears as an egg-shaped white region on the left of the figure. (B) MRI scan of a patient with a brain hemorrhage similar to that shown in (A). The area of bleeding is on the left of the figure and appears black on this image. (C) MRI scan showing a very large area of brain infarction on the left side of the figure. The infarct is white. This can be contrasted with the CT scan in Figure 8-1 in which the area of damage appears darker than the surrounding brain. (D) MRI scan showing a small infarct in the cerebellum on the left side of the figure. The white arrow points to the infarct, which appears white. On this scan, the right vertebral artery is seen as a round black area diagonally above the area of infarction. A small black arrow points to the vertebral artery.

the brain. *Magnetic resonance angiograms* (MRAs) can be made without injecting dye, by changing the settings on the MRI machine to capture vascular images instead of brain images. MRA can be performed at the same time as MRI; examinations using CTA can be done at the same time as CT. Figures 8-5 and 8-6 show examples of CTA and MRA images.

Ultrasound, sometimes called *Doppler* after Christian Doppler, who discovered the principle of ultrasound during his astronomy studies, is another very effective way to safely study blood flow in the arteries. This

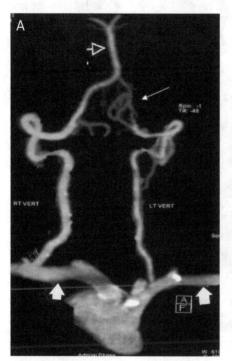
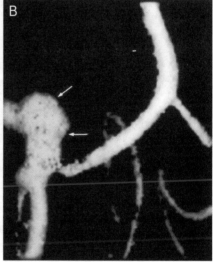

Figure 8-5

This figure shows two examples of CT angiograms (CTAs). (A) shows the subclavian arteries (large white arrowheads near the bottom of the figure. The vertebral arteries (marked right and left vertebral arteries) branch from the subclavian arteries and travel toward the brain. There is narrowing and irregularity of the left vertebral artery (long thin white arrow) after the artery enters the head. The two vertebral arteries join to form the basilar artery (open arrowhead). (B) shows a CTA of the vertebral and basilar arteries inside the head. A large aneurysm arises from the vertebral artery on the left (white arrows) The two vertebral arteries join to form the basilar artery as in (A).

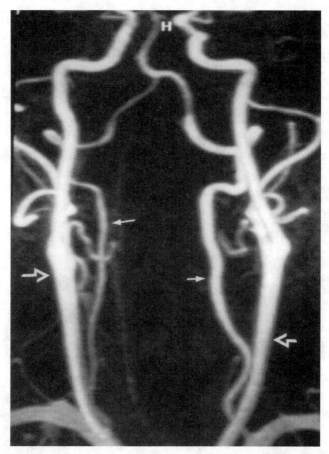

Figure 8-6

MRA showing all of the arteries that branch from the aorta going to the brain. The two open arrowheads on the outside of the arteries point to the carotid arteries. The two smaller white arrows on the inside point to the vertebral arteries.

type of testing is done by placing a small probe over blood vessels in the neck and over the eyes, back of the head, and sides of the head. The ultrasound information is relayed into an analyzing machine, which creates pictures of the vessels. The speed of the blood moving through the blood vessels directly under the probe is also calculated. Ultrasound findings can show if an artery is normal, narrowed, or completely blocked.

Duplex ultrasound scans of the neck create images and sound curves of the carotid and vertebral arteries in the neck. Figure 8-7A shows an

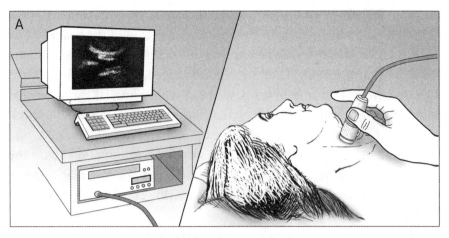

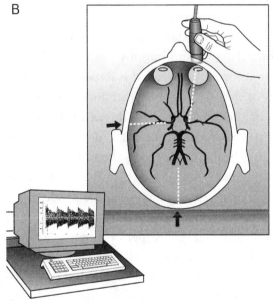

Figure 8-7

This figure shows an ultrasound examination; (A) shows an examination of the neck carotid artery and (B) shows a transcranial Doppler examination with the probe over the right eye.

example of an ultrasound examination of one carotid artery. Some laboratories use *transcranial* ultrasound (TCD) to examine blood flow in the arteries inside of the head. This technique is illustrated in Figure 8-7B. Using this technique, small probes are placed over the eyes, back of the neck, and temples. These are places where the skull is absent or thin. Blood flow velocities in the various arteries within the skull are also checked for narrowing, occlusion, or abnormally increased or decreased blood flow. When an artery in the neck is narrowed or blocked, TCD of the main branches of that artery in the head can reflect the impact of the neck disease on blood flow to the threatened region of the brain.

Single photon emission computed tomography (SPECT) is used to estimate blood flow to a region. After a chemical tagged with a radionuclide is injected into a vein, the brain is scanned with a special machine that detects the distribution of the injected substance. This helps identify relative blood flow to various parts of the brain, but, unlike MRA, CTA, and ultrasound, SPECT does not give images or direct information about the state of the supplying arteries. All of these brain and vascular imaging tests are quite safe and can be performed quickly either inside or outside the hospital.

When these so-called noninvasive tests do not give enough information about diseased arteries, physicians may order a *catheter angiogram*, which is performed by a specialist. This test is more invasive and carries a small but definite risk of complications. Doctors order this test when they judge that the information needed is important enough to warrant the small amount of risk. During this procedure, the specialist places a catheter in one of the arteries of the thighs or arms, and threads the catheter under visual control (using a TV monitoring fluoroscopic screen) into the arteries in the neck. Dye is then injected and a series of rapid-fire X-rays are taken that show the dye as it passes through the arteries and veins. This creates a picture of the inside of the arteries that can show areas of narrowing, blockage, aneurysms, and vascular malformations. At times, the specialist performing the angiography can give treatment to open narrowed or blocked arteries, or to obliterate vascular malformations or aneurysms.

Complications of catheter angiography most often consist of allergic response to the dye, inadvertent injury to the artery into which the catheter is placed, or dislodging of a plaque or clot from an artery that then passes into the brain. In the hands of well-trained and experienced specialists, these complications occur in only one or two patients in a hundred, and the great majority of complications are minor and temporary. Nevertheless, doctors try to avoid catheter angiography and most often rely on less invasive tests. The more the doctor knows about a patient's abnormalities, however, the better they can choose treatment.

Claire's MRA was normal, indicating that the embolus causing her symptoms and signs, and the brain infarct shown in Figure 8-2, had already passed through her blood vessels before the MRA was done. In contrast, Robert's MRA showed an occluded right internal carotid artery in his neck. A duplex ultrasound confirmed that his carotid artery was occluded. TCD showed low blood flow velocities over his right eye.

HEART TESTS

Heart testing is useful in almost all patients with stroke. The heart is often a source of clot formation. Clots and fragments of heart valves can

> Heart testing is useful in almost all patients with stroke.

break off and embolize to the brain, causing strokes. Individuals who have narrowing of the large arteries in the neck supplying blood to the brain often also have narrowing of the arteries supplying the heart muscle (the coronary arteries).

Electrocardiograms (EKGs) have long been used to study the heart. This test shows the rate at which the heart is beating (the pulse rate) and identifies abnormalities in the rhythm of the heart. This simple test can provide evidence of past heart attacks. Robert's electrocardiogram indicated a previous heart attack, but his heart rhythm was normal. Sam J. had atrial fibrillation confirmed on his electrocardiogram. Tom's EKG showed evidence of enlargement of the left-sided heart muscle (*left ventricular hypertrophy*) caused by his hypertension. Clair H. had a normal EKG.

Ultrasound of the heart (*echocardiography*) yields pictures of the various parts of the heart and their functioning. An *echocardiogram* is performed by a technician or a cardiologist by placing an ultrasound probe on the chest, or by having the patient swallow a string-like device containing an ultrasound probe into the esophagus. (Much of the heart is better seen from the back through the esophagus than from the front.) Using ultrasound, the cardiologist can see the heart valves, the upper heart chambers, and the left and right ventricles. Sometimes saline bubbles are injected into an arm vein so their passage through the heart can be observed. In Claire H., the injected bubbles passed from her right atrium into the left atrium through a hole in the wall (patent foramen ovale) between the two atria. Robert's echocardiogram showed a region of impaired contraction where he had had a myocardial infarct.

STUDYING THE ELECTRICAL ACTIVITY OF THE BRAIN

Doctors can record and study the electrical activity of the brain by placing small electrodes over the scalp. This test is called an *electroencephalogram* (EEG), and it is often used to distinguish between a transient ischemic attack (TIA) and a seizure arising from increased brain activity. Patients with seizures may have temporary interruptions in functioning that can be difficult to distinguish from TIAs without an EEG. Strokes can occasionally cause injuries that induce abnormal electrical discharge, causing patients to develop seizures.

BLOOD TESTS

Blood tests are routinely performed in patients who have had a stroke, or who are suspected of having a TIA or a stroke. The different types of blood tests are listed in Table 8-1. Of course, not all of these tests will be ordered for every patient.

> Blood tests are routinely performed in patients who have had a stroke.

Blood counts are routinely performed because overly high or low amounts of red and white blood cells and platelets can cause strokes and other medical problems. Screening tests of blood coagulation will be ordered—usually a prothrombin time and a platelet count. There will be further explorations of clotting abnormalities only when these screening tests are abnormal, or when there is a strong indication from the clini-

Table 8-1 Blood Tests

Blood counts
Red blood cells
Hemoglobin and hematocrit
White blood cells
Differential count of the various types of white blood cells (polymorphonuclear cells, lymphocytes, monocytes, eosinophils, basophils)
Platelets
Blood clotting tests
Prothrombin time (PT); often reported in terms of an International Normalized Ratio (INR)
Accelerated Partial Thromboplastin Time (APTT)
Antithrombin III, protein C, protein S
Factor V Leiden
Prothrombin gene mutation
Levels of blood factors II, VII, VIII, IX, X
Lupus anticoagulant, anticardiolipin antibodies
Blood sugar
Glycosylated hemoglobin- Hemoglobin A1C levels
Blood lipids
Total cholesterol
High and low-density lipoproteins (HDL and LDL)
Triglycerides
Lipoprotein a
Heart enzymes
Creatine kinase
cardiac (MB CK) and brain (BB CK) isoenzyme levels, troponin levels
Kidney function
Blood urea nitrogen (BUN)
Creatinine
Liver function
Bilirubin
Alkaline phosphatase
Blood electrolytes
Sodium
Potassium
Calcium
Chloride
Carbon dioxide (CO_2)
Homocysteine
Vitamin levels
B_{12}
Folic acid
Inflammatory markers and antibodies
Erythrocyte sedimentation rate (ESR)
C- reactive protein (CRP)
Fibrinogen
Antiphospholipid antibodies
Rheumatoid factor

cal history of excess clotting or excess bleeding. Most of the other tests will be selectively ordered, depending on the individual patient's risk factors, the nature of their stroke, and any coexisting medical conditions.

Most people are familiar with blood lipid tests, which are used to determine the levels of cholesterol, triglycerides, and other lipoproteins in the blood. High levels promote atherosclerosis and plaque formation in the arteries supplying the heart, brain, and limbs. Disorders of the kidneys, blood electrolytes, and the liver can cause or complicate strokes, and these factors are often measured in stroke patients. Cancers and a variety of inflammatory conditions can cause strokes. Thus, markers of inflammation and specific medical conditions are occasionally tested for in the blood.

Research has determined that elevated levels of homocysteine, CRP, and fibrinogen, and reduced levels of B_{12} predispose to stroke. These are often measured in patients thought to be at risk for stroke and/or heart disease and in those who have already had a stroke.

Centers specializing in stroke have technology and tests readily available. Individuals who are experienced in performing and interpreting the tests are on duty all of the time. Testing should be done quickly. Experienced neurologists can select the tests that are appropriate for each individual patient. Some tests need to be done quickly in patients with stroke; other tests can be ordered later. The brain is our most important resource, and it must be protected from stroke-related damage. The brain is vulnerable. Deprivation of necessary nutrients and oxygen can kill brain cells within minutes, or in only a few hours. The longer a brain region is deprived of normal blood flow, the more likely that region will die. The faster ischemia is corrected, the more chance there is of saving vital tissues. Whenever possible, patients must come to medical centers equipped to diagnose and treat them quickly, and doctors must pursue the investigations and treatment vigorously.

CHAPTER 9

What Treatments Are Available?

"You know that medicines when well used restore health to the sick. They will be well used when the doctor together with his understanding of their nature shall understand also what man is, what life is, and what constitution and health are."

Leonardo da Vinci

"One cannot possibly practice good medicine and not understand the fundamentals underlying therapy."

Dr. Fuller Albright

TREATMENT CHOICES FOR STROKE very much depend on the condition of the individual patient. Improved diagnostic technology, such as MRI, CT, and ultrasound, has made it much easier to precisely locate abnormalities and has greatly enhanced treatment. Medical, surgical, and radiologic techniques have been developed over the past three decades that greatly increase the ability of doctors to treat patients with brain hemorrhages and brain ischemia. It would be impossible in one chapter to capture the full details of treatment of stroke patients. I intend mostly to share the fundamental ideas on treatment (as Albright suggests in the quote at the beginning of the chapter). I have included some examples of the complexity of treatment decisions in individual patients at the end of this chapter.

ACUTE BRAIN ISCHEMIA

Three general treatment strategies are used in treating patients with an acute ischemic stroke:

- Increase blood flow as quickly as possible by opening blocked arteries
- Use medications to reduce the chances of formation and spread of blood clots
- Use medications that will make the vulnerable brain more resistant to damage from the ischemia

Opening Blocked Arteries

The most important strategy is to bring more blood to the threatened brain region. This tactic is called *reperfusion,* because it involves restoring blood flow to the regions of the brain that have recently been deprived of normal blood supply.

> The most important strategy is to bring more blood to the threatened brain region.

Consider this familiar situation as an analogy: watering a wilting lawn. Bringing blood to an ailing part of the brain is similar to bringing water to dry areas of a lawn. Assume the hose that supplies a portion of the lawn with water becomes blocked. A number of strategies can be used to restore the flow of water:

- You can try to unblock the hose by cutting it open and removing the obstruction (a surgical procedure called *endarterectomy*).
- You can use a mechanical instrument to unblock the hose (*angioplasty*).
- After successful unblocking, you might want to place a mechanical layer within the hose to strengthen it (*stenting*) to make sure the hose does not become blocked again.
- You can introduce a chemical compound to dissolve whatever is blocking the hose (*thrombolysis*).
- Alternatively, if you are not able to remove or dissolve the obstruction, you can create a detour around the blockage by attaching another piece of hose to the segment of the hose *before* the blocked area and attaching it beyond the region of blockage (*surgical bypass*).

Thrombolysis

Doctors use the types of strategies described above in patients with acute ischemic strokes who have blockage in arteries. *Thrombolysis* is the term used to describe chemical dissolution of clots that are blocking arteries. The most common *thrombolytic* medication used, and the only acute stroke drug now approved by the Federal Drug Authority (FDA), is *tissue plasminogen activator* (t-PA). Researchers are exploring other potential agents. T-PA and other thrombolytic medications can be given either intravenously or by having a specialist place a catheter within the blocked artery to deliver the medication directly to the clot. To be effective, t-PA must be given soon after stroke symptoms develop. The side effects of thrombolytic medications include bleeding into the brain and other organs. The bleeding can be serious and even fatal.

Thrombolysis is hazardous when the blood pressure is very high, when the patient's blood clotting system indicates a tendency for bleeding, and when the patient has had recent surgery or another type of intervention. Thrombolysis is not appropriate for every patient who is seen soon after stroke, but every patient seen by physicians soon after stroke onset should be carefully evaluated to determine if this treatment is appropriate for him. The risk of treatment may outweigh the potential benefit when extensive brain infarction is already present and when arteries are not blocked. Whether or not to use t-PA and other thrombolytic medications is a decision based on the doctor's judgment, and depends on a number of different considerations. The potential risks and benefits of this and other treatments should be discussed with the patients and their families.

Surgery

If they are able to expose the blocked artery segment, in the neck, surgeons can operate directly on an artery to try and unblock it. This procedure is called an *endarterectomy*, because the inner portion of the artery (*endartery*) is removed. A temporary clamp is placed above and below the diseased segment, and then the artery is opened and the inner core of plaque and clot material is removed. After the artery has been cleaned out, it is sewed back up and the clamps are removed. This process takes a half-hour or less in most cases. Endarterectomies are usually feasible when the artery is severely narrowed but not totally blocked. It is usually performed to prevent future strokes as opposed to treating a stroke that has already developed. Clots sometimes block an artery and extend far beyond their origin, making it impossible to reopen the artery surgically. Endarterectomy is used almost entirely for blockage within the neck—the carotid and vertebral arteries. Most of the arteries that commonly block within the head are not readily exposed for surgery.

If the blocked arteries cannot be repaired directly, surgeons can reconstruct the blood flow channels by using various techniques. Part of the artery can be tied into another artery toward the head. Alternatively, they can bring another artery into a position next to the blocked artery and sew the two vessels together, or they can take a loop of another vessel from a distant site and use it to detour around the blocked artery. Doctors sometimes place a muscle or tissue from the abdomen onto the outside of the brain in an ischemic area and sew the tissue to the surface in an effort to encourage ingrowth of blood vessels from the tissue into the brain. This technique is used most frequently in an unusual disorder that affects young people called *Moya Moya syndrome*. In this condition, the carotid arteries inside the skull and their large artery branches gradually become blocked, and blood flow to the brain becomes severely compromised.

Angioplasty and Stenting

Using an option called *angioplasty*, an instrument can be inserted within an artery to dilate (open) it. This technique can be used to open arteries within the neck and head, especially when those arteries are not readily accessible for surgery. Sometimes doctors use a *stent* after angioplasty to keep the artery open, or they may put in a stent without doing an angioplasty first. Stents are mechanical sleeves that expand to dilate the lumen of an artery and keep it open wide. The stents remain in place to keep the artery open.

Opening Narrowed Carotid Arteries

Atherosclerosis in the internal carotid artery in the neck is very common, especially in white men. When an individual develops a TIA or minor stroke in the territory of supply of a carotid artery that is >70% narrowed, the risk of stroke if untreated is very high. The risk of stroke is about 30 to 35% in the near future. Carotid endarterectomy decreases the stroke risk in these symptomatic patients. The surgery may not be appropriate after a large stroke. If six or seven patients have carotid surgery, one stroke will be prevented. Carotid artery angioplasty and stenting have recently been approved for patients who have a high risk for surgery. Research trials are now occurring to compare the effectiveness and safety of carotid artery stenting as compared with surgery.

More controversial is carotid endarterectomy and carotid artery stenting in patients with carotid artery narrowing who have never had a related stroke or TIA. Large trials show some benefit in very selected patients with severe carotid artery narrowing who have been operated on by very selected surgeons. The risk of developing a stroke in patients who have no ischemic symptoms related to the narrowed artery is about 2 to 2.5% a year. The risk of stroke or death with the surgery varies between 1 and 5% depending on the surgeon and the disease severity of the patients. A surgeon would have to perform 70 to 90 surgeries in asymptomatic patients to prevent one stroke. Carotid stents are now also being studied as an alternative to surgical carotid endarterectomy.

Maximizing Blood Flow

It is important to improve blood flow to the head. When an artery is blocked, blood flow to the ischemic zone and its surrounding tissues comes from other nearby arteries (called *collateral channels*), which ordinarily do not directly supply that region. Ischemic brain tissue produces

> It is important to improve blood flow to the head.

chemicals that encourage ingrowth of collateral blood vessels to help make up for the lack of blood flow. Doctors may try to boost this process by maintaining or slightly increasing blood pressure, increasing the amount of fluid in the body, and decreasing the viscosity (actual thickness) of the blood. Lowering blood pressure can increase blood flow in patients with very high blood pressure. Treating high blood sugar may also help normalize energy delivery.

Changing the Tendency of Blood to Clot

Another common strategy often used in patients with vessel narrowing or occlusion, or embolism, is to use various medications that reduce the body's tendency to form clots. These medications are classified as *anticoagulants* and *antiplatelet agents*. The purpose of using these medications is to prevent formation of blood clots in the heart and the aorta, and in regions of vascular narrowing and irregularity. Brain ischemia is caused by vascular occlusion, and blood clotting plays a crucial role in blocking the vessels. Of course, giving an agent that will reduce the coagulability of the blood is potentially disastrous if the stroke is due to hemorrhage.

Two different types of agents are used to alter blood coagulability. Antiplatelet agents primarily alter the function of blood platelets. When an artery becomes irregular and a plaque forms, the altered inner lining of the blood vessel stimulates platelets in the blood to stick to the surface of the plaque and to stick together. This creates a small white clot made of platelets and fibrin. The fibrin comes from a circulating serum protein-fibrinogen. The white clot can subsequently be displaced from the vessel and can embolize to vessels within the brain, causing TIAs and strokes. Activation of platelets can also stimulate the formation of a superimposed red clot made of red blood cells admixed with fibrin. One strategy to discourage platelet agglutination and adhesion is to give medications that decrease these platelet functions. Aspirin, clopidogrel, dipyridamole, and cilostazole are the best known antiplatelet agents. The medications are sometimes combined together into one pill, for example, aspirin with modified release dipyridamole. Most of the nonsteroidal medications used for arthritis and pain relief also have antiplatelet actions; these medications include ibuprofen and indomethacin. Some natural food substances, such as omega-3 oils derived from fish and the black tree fungus found in many Chinese foods, are rich in substances that effect platelet functions. These antiplatelet medicines are most often used to prevent future strokes.

One relatively new class of antiplatelet agents affects the attachment of platelets to fibrinogen. These medications are called *GP llb/llla inhibitors*. The most commonly used such medication is abciximab (Reopro®), which is given only intravenously in acute situations when white platelet-fibrin clots are thought to block arteries. Unfortunately, the use of these agents is sometimes accompanied by bleeding. Research is exploring similar medications that can be given intravenously or by mouth.

Another strategy is to give anticoagulants, which lessen the tendency for red clots to form. Although these medications are often referred to as "blood thinners," they really do not change the thickness and viscosity of the blood. Rather, they make the blood flowing in the vessels less likely to clot. A natural substance called *heparin*, or similar substances called *heparinoids*, or low-molecular-weight heparins, are often given by injection or intravenously while stroke patients are in the hospital. Later, warfarin-type medications, including coumadin, are given by mouth. The activity of coumadin depends on its influence in decreasing the effect of prothrombin. A side effect of coumadin is that it decreases the clotting tendency of the blood, making spontaneous bleeding and bleeding after a cut or injury a potential problem.

In order to monitor the tendency of the blood to clot in patients taking warfarin-type anticoagulants, doctors order blood tests to compare the patient's tendency to clot against normal standards. These tests are called *prothrombin time determinations*. The results are given in time (14 seconds); in a ratio of the patient's prothrombin time to local controls in that lab (2 times control); or as a ratio determined by comparison with an international standard, the INR (International Normalized Ratio) (2.1 INR). The blood must be monitored frequently, at first, to make sure that the results show enough lessening of clotting tendency without excessive risk of bleeding. Usually, the physician or a nurse or laboratory assistant will call the patient after the test and tell the patient how many pills to take that day and on subsequent days, and when to have the next blood test.

Blood coagulability and the effectiveness of coumadin are changed by many other medications and by some foods. Coumadin dosage is also affected by hormonal fluctuations in women, such as menstruation, pregnancy, ovulation, use of oral contraceptives, and female hormones used for any reason. Some of the other factors that can alter the dose of coumadin and its effects are not known.

A new type of anticoagulant has recently been introduced into medical care. These agents, including ximelagatran and argatraban, have a direct effect on thrombin. They do not work on prothrombin as warfarin does. Unlike warfarin compounds, the dose of the direct thrombin inhibitors does not change, and tests are not needed to monitor the extent of the effect on blood clotting. Ximelagatran is taken as a pill twice a day; argatraban has to be given intravenously.

Neuroprotective Agents

Another relatively new treatment strategy to try to prevent or at least diminish brain ischemia is to give various medications that reduce the vulnerability of the tissues to ischemia. These medications are usually referred to as *neuroprotective agents*. Returning to the wilting lawn analogy, the use of neuroprotective agents can be likened to sprinkling something on the grass that would somehow make it more resistant to wilting during a drought. Neuroprotection is a new strategy, and many medications and physical measures are being studied. These medications can be given to patients with ischemia or threatened ischemia immediately after the first symptoms appear. The use of these medications might give treating physicians a little more time to accomplish reperfusion and still preserve threatened brain tissue.

Another strategy that is being tested is cooling the body and brain to below normal body temperature (*hypothermia*). This strategy has been used in the past during heart and brain surgery. When organs are at a lower than normal temperature, they require less energy to sustain them. It is hoped that the reduced blood supply will be enough to take care of the reduced energy demands.

Treating Acute Hemorrhage

Treatment of bleeding inside of the head is more simple and direct than the complicated and multifaceted treatment of the different aspects of brain ischemia. Aneurysms that cause sudden bleeding in the membranes surrounding the brain (*subarachnoid hemorrhage*) can be clipped during surgery to prevent a second episode of bleeding. At times, aneurysms and vascular malformations can be obliterated by catheters placed within the feeding arteries through which various coils and other substances can be delivered to correct the vascular abnormalities. Vascular malformations can also sometimes be removed surgically or obliterated by focused radiation. Doctors may be able to drain brain hemorrhages using surgery when they are large and threaten life. Reduction of blood pressure and reversal of any tendency for excess bleeding can also be used to try to limit further hemorrhaging into the brain. This is especially important in patients taking warfarin (coumadin), as their bleeding tendency can be reversed by infusing into their veins clotting factors contained in fresh frozen plasma. Trials are now underway to test whether giving potent clotting factors will be able to safely stop bleeding into the brain.

THERAPEUTIC TRIALS

Therapeutic trials have helped doctors learn much about treatment. When there is no proven effective treatment for a condition, a therapeutic trial studies treatment with a medicine and compares the results with treatment using a placebo (a "sugar pill" not known to have any effect on the condition being studied). When one or more treatments are already known to be effective for a specific condition, a trial considers a new treatment compared with already recognized treatments. An example of this type of trial is comparing carotid artery stenting with carotid surgery among patients in whom carotid artery surgery has already been proven to be effective. In therapeutic trials, the effectiveness and safety of the treatments are analyzed. Which treatment a given individual receives is chose at random; the randomization process is like a flip of a coin—heads results in one treatment, tails another. Most often neither the doctors giving the treatment nor the patients receiving the treatments are aware of which treatment is being given ("double-blind"). The reason for blinding both doctors and patients is the very strong hope and conviction that both share that their favored treatment should work (and the placebo or other treatment should not work).

The results of therapeutic trials have helped doctors recognize that:

- Individuals who have atrial fibrillation have much less chance of developing a stroke if they are treated with anticoagulants such as warfarin (coumadin) compared to treatment with no anticoagulant or aspirin.
- Individuals who have severe narrowing of their carotid arteries in the neck, and who develop symptoms explained by reduced blood flow in the eye or brain tissue supplied by the narrowed artery, have less strokes when carotid artery surgery is performed by experienced surgeons who have a low rate of complications.
- Older individuals who have high systolic blood pressures have fewer strokes when treated with antihypertensive medicines than patients who are not given antihypertensive treatments.
- Individuals with acute strokes have less brain damage when treated with rt-PA given intravenously during the first three hours after stroke onset than those patients not given rt-PA.
- Aspirin, clopidogrel, and aspirin combined with modified-release dipyridamole are effective in preventing strokes in individuals who have had TIAs or minor strokes.

It is very important for individuals to understand what therapeutic trials are and how they are conducted. The public and individuals should recognize that trials are the very best way to scientifically study the effectiveness and safety of various treatments. Many treatments have been proposed and vigorously supported by physicians and researchers alike, but these treatments have later been shown to be ineffective and sometimes dangerous when therapeutic trials have been performed. Whenever available, join a trial rather than accept a treatment not proven to be effective.

Some Examples of Difficult Treatment Decisions

Even when trials have shown that a treatment is generally effective among a large number of patients, it might not be wise to use it in a given situation in a particular individual. Patients are all different. They have different disease burdens and different past experiences. Their wishes and hopes and fears also may be quite different. Some individuals, when told the potential risks and benefits of a treatment, might accept that treatment while others given the same information would not. Some patients and their families are very conservative and some are risk-takers. Decisions need to be made with full cooperation between doctor and patient. A few examples will illustrate the complexity of some treatment decisions.

Jerome H., a 78-year-old man, suddenly developed slurred speech and slight clumsiness of his right hand. He had been healthy in the past, other than coronary artery disease and slight hypertension, well-controlled with medicines, He had been taking 40 mg of a statin and one 325 mg aspirin a day on the advice of his doctor. His wife took him quickly to a stroke center for treatment and he arrived two hours after the onset of his stroke symptoms. The doctors performed a head CT scan and a CT angiogram. These studies showed that he had had two very small minor areas of damage in the left cerebral hemisphere supplied by the left carotid artery. The left carotid artery in the neck was narrowed by >75%. There was no blockage of any artery inside of the head.

The doctors decided not to give the patient rt-PA. Instead they gave him heparin. Five days later, at which time he had recovered normal speech and very good hand function, they performed a left carotid endarterectomy. He left the hospital without any important handicap.

At first Jerome's wife and family did not understand why rt-PA was not given when he first arrived. They had heard about rt-PA and had struggled to bring him to the hospital as soon as possible. The doctors explained to the family that even though he had arrived within three hours, his deficit was slight; the potential risk of bleeding outweighed the gain of giving rt-PA, since good recovery was expected without its use. The doctors also discussed the fact that the only function of rt-PA is to break down clots that are blocking arteries. The CTA had shown that there were no clots in the main arteries. Any clot material that had formed had already passed through the brain circulation. In Jerome's case, the best treatment was to prevent new clots from forming by giving heparin. Then prevention of new strokes could best be accomplished by performing carotid artery surgery. There was a long discussion concerning the choice of surgery as opposed to carotid artery stenting. After weighing the risks and benefits, the family chose the surgical option.

Richard P., a 36-year-old healthy man was noted by his wife to be snoring loudly. His wife attempted to awaken him, but she could not arouse him. She called 911, and an ambulance took him to a stroke center. Doctors found that he did not respond when they spoke to him or tried to arouse him. His left limbs were paralyzed. His eyes looked far to the right side. A CT scan showed a very large infarct involving almost the entire portion of the brain supplied by the right carotid artery. A CTA showed a dissection of the carotid artery in the neck. When the findings were discussed with the wife, she recalled that he had had a minor neck injury while playing soccer a week ago and that he had told her about headaches during the past few days.

The doctors did not give Richard rt-PA. They explained to his wife that there was no way of knowing when the stroke had developed and how long the brain had been deprived of energy. Furthermore, nearly all the brain tissue fed by the blocked artery had already been irreversibly damaged. There was no remaining tissue to save. Giving rt-PA would also carry a great risk for bleeding into the dead brain tissue.

When Richard became completely comatose that afternoon, the doctors discussed with his wife whether or not they should pursue aggressive life-saving procedures. Would Richard want to continue to live if he had severe left limb paralysis? Had he ever discussed his feelings about aggressive invasive treatment were he to develop a potentially disabling medical condition?

Richard's wife Ellen had never discussed these issues with her husband. He was young and healthy, and Ellen thought that everything should be done. A neurosurgeon removed a large portion of the skull on the right side of Richard's head so that the brain would not be compressed and further damaged by pressure against the skull bones. This procedure is called a *hemicraniectomy*, a term that literally means removing skull bone on one half of the head. One week after the surgery, Richard began to awaken. After a long stay in a rehabilitation hospital, he returned home and was able to walk. His left limbs remained paralyzed, but he was happy to still be alive. With determination and time he was able to return to work at his former job in a convenience store very near his home.

Rachel L., a 51-year-old nurse suddenly during dinner became unable to move her left arm and leg. She had been quite healthy but recently had noticed that her pulse sometimes became rapid and irregular. She had called to make an appointment with her doctor but had not seen her as yet. An ambulance took Rachel to the nearest hospital, where they performed an electrocardiogram that showed that Rachel had atrial fibrillation. They performed a CT scan that was interpreted as normal. Because they were not a stroke center and felt poorly equipped to treat Rachel, they decided to send her by another ambulance to a stroke center in town. Rachel arrived at the academic stroke center four hours after her stroke symptoms began.

Another CT scan showed a small region of infarction in the right cerebral hemisphere and a bright right middle cerebral artery, indicating that a clot was present in that artery. The diagnosis was clear. Rachel had developed a clot in her atrium as a result of the atrial fibrillation. The clot had embolized to her right middle cerebral artery, causing the left limb paralysis. The doctors gave her rt-PA intravenously. Almost immediately, Rachel began to move her left arm and leg although it remained slightly weak.

Unfortunately an hour later the left limbs again became paralyzed. After discussion with the family, the doctors called in a specialist to perform a cerebral arteriogram. This showed that the clot had reformed in the right middle cerebral artery and was blocking blood flow. The specialist directed a catheter into the right middle cerebral artery and infused a thrombolytic drug, urokinase. The artery partially opened. The specialist then placed a mechanical retrieval device that looked like a paper clip into the catheter and directed it towards the clot. He was able to snag the clot using the device and to bring it down the catheter all the way out of Rachel's body. He instilled some dye and took a picture that showed that the middle cerebral artery and all its branches were now fully open. After the procedure Rachel was able to move her left arm and leg well, and within two days she left the hospital without any noticeable injury. Because of her atrial fibrillation, Rachel's doctors prescribed coumadin to prevent clots from forming again in her heart.

Many lessons can be gleaned from Rachel's story:

- If symptoms that suggest heart problems develop, such as a fast or irregular heart beat, you must see a doctor as soon as possible.
- When symptoms of a stroke or TIA develop be sure to go to the nearest stroke center. Do not allow an ambulance to take you or your loved one to a hospital that is not equipped to handle stroke unless there is no alternative and no stroke center is available anywhere nearby. Go to the most advanced stroke center as quickly as possible. Before an emergency occurs, find out where in your area is the best place to go to treat a heart attack and stroke.
- Although the media has popularized the three hour rule for rt-PA, the decision whether to give the drug in an individual situation and when is more complex than looking at a watch. Patients do not automatically change from good candidates to no candidate when the clock strikes three. Some patients seen within three hours should not get rt-PA. Some patients seen after three hours, like Rachel L., are good candidates. The decision is complex and is best made by experienced doctors at stroke centers that have the best equipment and personnel to evaluate stroke patients.
- There are a number of ways to try to dissolve clots or remove them other than by giving rt-PA by vein. Specialists can administer thrombolytic drugs directly into an artery that is blocked and can use a number of mechanical retrievers to attempt to remove the clot. Research is exploring new throbolytic drugs and new mechanical devices.

PREVENTING ANOTHER STROKE

Prevention is always preferred to treatment after the fact. Chapters 3 and 4 reviewed various medical conditions and risk factors that predis-

Prevention is always preferred to treatment after the fact.

pose people to develop strokes. Prevention was also discussed. These same principles of prevention also apply to preventing further strokes in patients who have already had a stroke (secondary prevention). Some of the most important prevention strategies include:

Hypertension Control

Different methods can be used to reduce elevated blood pressure. Losing weight and exercise are clearly quite effective in many patients. Reducing salt intake is also useful. A variety of different medications can be prescribed. (Table 4-2 lists some of the classes of medications and the commonly used medications in each class.) Often it becomes necessary to use more than one medication to adequately control high blood pressure.

Diabetes Control

Exercise and weight loss in individuals who are overweight are effective and important interventions in diabetic individuals. When, how much, and what you eat are also important. A variety of medications can be used to reduce blood sugar (Table 4-3). Patients who have very low levels of insulin can be treated by injections of different types of insulin, sometimes more than once a day.

Controlling Elevated Levels of Blood Lipids

Reduction of high cholesterol and triglyceride levels is an important goal. Many patients can achieve this result by diet management. In oth-

Reduction of high cholesterol and triglyceride levels is an important goal.

ers, use of a statin medication, such as simvastatin, atorvastatin, or pravastatin, is very effective in reducing total cholesterol levels. It has been shown that statins reduce plaque formation and stroke in patients who have arterial plaques and narrowing, even when their cholesterol levels are normal. Statins have a good effect on the lining of blood vessels in addition to their effect on blood cholesterol. (The common medications used to lower blood lipids are also listed in Table 4-4.)

Use of Anticoagulants and Antiplatelets

As discussed previously, antiplatelets and anticoagulants are used in preventing first and subsequent strokes, as well as in acute ischemic stroke. Anticoagulants (both warfarin compounds and direct thrombin inhibitors) have been used to prevent stroke in patients such as Sam J., who had atrial fibrillation. Antiplatelet agents have been shown to be very effective in stroke prevention in patients who have stroke risk factors, and in those individuals who have had a TIA or minor stroke.

Changing Unhealthy Lifestyles

Smoking and heavy use of alcohol are well established risk factors for stroke as well as other serious medical diseases. Stopping smoking is essential for anyone who has had a stroke or who has risk factors for stroke. One or two drinks of alcohol a day has not been shown to be harmful, but heavier drinking definitely poses a risk for stroke. Every effort should be made to stop smoking and moderate excess drinking of alcohol. Other life-style changes, such as loss of excess weight and increase in physical activity level, are strongly encouraged.

CHAPTER 10

What Are the Complications of Stroke?

"The best laid plans of mice and men often go astray."

Robert Burns

S TROKES CAN BE FOLLOWED by a host of other problems, as can many other serious medical illnesses. I have often heard family members say, "Mom was okay when she got to the hospital with a stroke, but then complications set in." Complications may occur during hospitalization for acute stroke, or they may develop during rehabilitation and during subsequent neurologic recovery.

There are three general types of complications:

- Neurologic, causing brain function to worsen
- Medical, involving organs other than the brain
- Psychologic—strokes are often followed by depression

NEUROLOGIC COMPLICATIONS

Worsening of Brain Ischemia

Brain function may deteriorate during the first hours and days in the hospital, despite even the best medical treatment. Doctors characterize this worsening as "progressing stroke." Patients may enter the hospital with only minor symptoms, and then hours or days later develop quite severe loss of brain functions because of progression of their strokes. Minor weakness of the left arm and leg can progress to total paralysis of those limbs.

> Brain function may deteriorate during the
> first hours and days in the hospital, despite
> even the best medical treatment.

The worsening is often due to continuation of the process that originally caused the stroke. Bleeding can continue in patients with hemorrhages. Recall Tom M., the 41-year-old longshoreman with hypertension and a drinking problem, who developed a hemorrhage into his brain—an intracerebral hemorrhage. When he came to the hospital, he had a headache, felt dizzy, and staggered when he walked. CT scans showed that he had a hemorrhage in the cerebellum (Figure 8-3). His condition worsened during the first hours in the hospital, and a repeat CT scan showed that the hemorrhage had grown larger. Patients who are hospitalized because of a subarachnoid hemorrhage due to a ruptured aneurysm may rebleed during the hospitalization before doctors can repair the aneurysm.

Ischemic strokes are caused by an insufficient blood supply to a part of the brain. The insufficiency can persist and lead to a gradual or stepwise loss of brain function. For example, recall Robert H., the patient with an occlusion of a carotid artery in his neck. A clot within the carotid artery can extend or embolize, causing further brain damage. If the source of the embolus in the heart, aorta, or large artery is not controlled in patients with brain embolism, they can throw off another embolus, causing further brain damage.

Brain Edema

Another important cause of worsening during the acute stroke period is brain edema and swelling. Injured tissue often induces a reaction around its perimeter that stimulates a pouring out of tissue fluid. Brain hemorrhages and brain infarcts often become surrounded by an accumulation of fluid, referred to as *brain edema*. Recall an instance when you have hit an arm or a leg, creating a bruise. The area around the bruised tissue probably swelled up during the hours and days after the injury. Edema fluid naturally develops after a brain injury. The swollen tissue compresses nearby structures and is often accompanied by headache, worsening of the neurologic deficit, and a decrease in the level of alertness. Doctors can prescribe medicines to draw the fluid out of the brain.

Seizures

Seizures are not a common complication of stroke, but they do occur. Those that occur in stroke patients are usually relatively easy to control with medication. The brain is an electrical organ made up of millions of nerve cells that transmit messages electrically at synapses. The electrical activity of these cells is normally related to activity in the environment and inside the body. A seizure can be thought of as a type of inappropriate activity or short circuit in a part of the brain during which some nerve cells discharge spontaneously and hyperactively. The nerve cells that discharge have been partially damaged by brain ischemia or hemorrhage. These injured cells can discharge repeatedly, even in the absence of an appropriate stimulus. A simple analogy is a failing light bulb. When some of the light bulb filaments are worn out, they will spontaneously light up for a moment and flicker uncontrollably, even when the switch is turned off. Similarly, partially damaged nerve cells can discharge even when they are not stimulated.

Excessive discharge of local neurons sometimes quickly spreads throughout the nervous system and a seizure occurs. Seizures can take many forms. They can be convulsive, causing violent contractions of the muscles of the limbs, face, and jaw. Often, the muscles stiffen before

Seizures can take many forms.

they rhythmically jerk. Pelvic and abdominal muscle contractions can cause a release of urine and bowel contents during a seizure. Patients are unconscious during a seizure, and afterwards they usually do not recall the attack. Seizure sometimes spreads to both sides of the brain. These patients look blank and momentarily lose consciousness, but do not shake. The discharge remains local in some patients, who develop localized jerking of muscles on their weak side. This local discharge may cause a visual, tactile, auditory, or olfactory experience, or an inappropriate emotional reaction.

When seizures complicate strokes, most often they develop after the acute stroke period, when some nerve cells have partially recovered. An initial seizure is often very alarming to observers, although patients are most often unaware of what happens during the seizure. Often, seizures are followed by a period of drowsiness and decreased alertness. The nerve cells, having discharged vigorously, have used up a good deal of energy and require time to recover. Headache, tired aching muscles, and a bitten tongue are often present after motor seizures as a result of increased muscle activity during the seizure. Patients report that their muscles feel as if they had been beaten up, or as if they had run vigorously. After a seizure, patients sometimes become temporarily violent and strike out at individuals who are trying to help them. They often recognize that they have had a seizure because of a gap in their recall of events, or because of the feelings in their muscles, their sore tongue, and the evidence of incontinence, which they see when they awaken after the seizure.

Seizures almost always stop spontaneously. Observers need not stick anything in a person's mouth during a seizure. The idea of swallowing the tongue is a myth. The seizing individual should be placed on a soft bed, if possible, or at least in a place where they will not injure themselves during the shaking. They should be taken to a hospital if it is their first seizure. Otherwise, they need not be taken to a hospital after a seizure, unless the seizures are repetitive, or if they do not wake up within 10 to 15 minutes. The treating doctor should be notified later so that medications can be adjusted if necessary.

MEDICAL COMPLICATIONS

Pneumonia

Stroke patients often develop pneumonia in the hospital. A number of different factors related to stroke predispose a patient to the develop-

Stroke patients often develop pneumonia in the hospital.

ment of lung infection. Strokes often cause weakness of the structures within the mouth and throat that relate to the swallowing of solids and liquids. As a result, food and saliva within the mouth can go down the wrong way. Instead of proceeding from the mouth to the esophagus to the stomach, the swallowed substances can go into the larynx and from there into the lungs. This is called *aspiration*. Many different bacteria live in the mouth and, of course, foods are not sterile. As a result, infected material can reach the lungs and cause pneumonia.

Another factor that makes stroke patients susceptible to pneumonia relates to breathing functions after stroke. Individuals whose left arm and leg become weak may also have some weakness of the chest muscles on the left side that move air into the left lung. The left lung is underventilated, especially in bed. It is much easier to take a deep breath if you are sitting or standing, rather than lying flat in bed. Areas within the lung that are not well filled with air become more susceptible to infection. Stroke patients with weakness also may have difficulty coughing and clearing their airways of mucus and aspirated substances.

Doctors try to prevent pneumonia in stroke patients who have difficulty swallowing by not feeding them by mouth. Sitting up in bed and breathing deeply will also help prevent the development of pneumonia. Early antibiotic treatment when pneumonia does develop is also important.

Urinary Tract Infection

Strokes often affect the mechanics of urination. Retention of urine and difficulty in voluntarily emptying the bladder are common accompaniments of stroke. Passing urine is also more difficult in bed than sitting on a toilet or, for men, standing. Compounding urinary difficulty is the fact that most stroke-age men have enlarged prostate glands, and have previously had some difficulty in urinating, even before their strokes. The tissues around the urinary passages in the pelvis are not sterile. Infection very often develops when urine remains pooled in the bladder. Bacterial infections within the urinary system can reach the kidneys, and can also enter the blood stream.

Another common cause of urinary infections is the presence of an indwelling urinary catheter. Catheters are often inserted into the bladder of stroke patients who cannot urinate or who become incontinent. Bacteria have an easy entry into the bladder along these catheters. Leaving a catheter inside the bladder is more likely to lead to a urinary tract infection than intermittent catheterization.

Thrombophlebitis and Pulmonary Embolism

Stroke patients are prone to developing blood clots within their legs, especially in limbs that are weak. These blood clots can travel to the lungs and cause pulmonary embolism, a life-threatening condition. Motion of the limbs and contraction of the muscles within the limbs keeps blood circulating in the veins. When stroke causes paralysis of the muscles in one leg, and the leg is not moved normally, the stasis of blood predisposes to clot formation. Also, many strokes cause activation of the blood clotting system, a factor that also predisposes to clot formation.

A number of strategies are used to prevent clotting within the legs. Early walking and mobilization are important. Special stockings that help move blood along in the legs are also often used. Doctors usually prescribe an anticoagulant, such as heparin, to patients who are not mobile. Heparin is given in small doses by injection as a clot preventative measure.

Myocardial Infarction ("Heart Attack")

Heart and brain vascular disease often coexist. Cardiac dysfunction is another frequent accompaniment of stroke. A dysfunctioning heart may be the source of stroke, it may coexist with stroke, or it may be caused by the stroke. Many individuals who have disease of the arteries supplying the brain also have disease of the arteries supplying the heart.

Heart and brain vascular disease often coexist.

Atherosclerosis is a condition that can affect many arteries. Heart attacks can precede a stroke. In this case, a clot has often formed within the ventricle of the heart and embolized to the brain, causing the stroke. The preceding heart attack may not be diagnosed until after the stroke occurs.

Stroke precedes the heart attack in some patients. As mentioned in the discussion of thrombophlebitis and pulmonary embolism, strokes can activate the body's coagulation system. This activation can cause clot formation in already narrowed coronary arteries, leading to a heart attack.

Bed Sores

Stroke patients with reduced mobility who cannot reposition themselves, and do not sense the need to change position, are at risk of developing bedsores if they are not frequently turned and repositioned. Incontinence wets the skin with an acidic fluid (urine), increasing the risk of developing skin breakdown. Prevention of skin ulceration is very important in stroke patients who have paralysis. Early mobilization is necessary, and stroke patients should be turned frequently. The skin should be kept clean and dry. Adequate nutrition should be given. Pressure on arms and legs that have reduced sensation and on immobilized limbs must be avoided. The use of padded heel boots can spare the heels from ulcers. Egg-crate mattresses, waterbeds, and soft cotton padding may help prevent the development of sacral pressure sores on or near the buttocks. Nurses often periodically check the entire surface of a patient's body to look for any area of early skin breakdown. Particular attention should be paid to susceptible areas, such as the buttock, heels, elbows, wrists, between the toes, and the back of the head. If an ulcer develops, pressure on that area should be totally avoided, special mattresses should be used, and the wound should be dressed. If necessary, damaged tissue can be surgically removed to facilitate healing.

Contractures and Shoulder Pain

Immobility of the limbs and maintenance in fixed, usually flexed positions can lead to fixed contractures at the knees and elbows. Decreased shoulder movement can lead to shoulder pain, frozen shoulders, and swelling of the hand and forearm. The weight of a paralyzed arm hanging in a downward position can cause the arm bone (the *humerus*) to pop out of the shoulder joint. The weak arm should not be left to hang without support. Severe shoulder weakness and dislocation of the shoulder increase the likelihood of developing shoulder pain and swelling of the arm. Early full range of movement of the shoulder joint is very important in preventing this unpleasant and disabling stroke complication. Physical therapists can teach patients and caregivers how to keep the affected shoulder mobile, even when the arm is weak.

Osteoporosis

Studies of bone density after stroke show that there is a reduction in bone mineral density on the paralyzed side. Calcium removal from immobilized bone, lack of exposure to sunlight, poor nutrition with inadequate Vitamin D stores, and osteoporosis before the stroke increase osteoporosis after stroke. Osteoporosis is the most severe in patients with severe paralysis, especially those who have prolonged immobilization. The reduced bone density of osteoporosis predisposes patients to hip and other fractures, which tend to occur mostly on the paralyzed side. Early mobilization, exposure to sunlight, and giving calcium and vitamin D supplements can prevent or minimize this stroke complication.

Depression and Other Psychologic Reactions

The reactions of patients to their strokes vary. New personality traits can emerge, and old ones become accentuated after stroke. Some patients see the stroke as a "wake-up-call." They fight vigorously to return to their normal activities and pay more attention to their health and lifestyle than they did before their stroke. They view the stroke as a kind of blessing that awakened them to pursue better health. Some become

New personality traits can emerge and old ones become accentuated after stroke.

angry at what they feel is unfair "punishment." They ask, "Why did God do this to me?" They reason that they did nothing to deserve their handicap. Others, who had ignored their own risk factors, feel guilty and upset with themselves for not being more health conscious, and for not listening to their doctor. Many feel guilty at placing a burden on their spouses and other caregivers.

Some stroke patients become depressed and feel hopeless about the future. One of the most important and yet most frequently overlooked complications of stroke is depression. Family members often report that the patient is no longer particularly weak, and is able to get around well, but they are not acting normally. Dependency and lack of social contacts are important factors in promoting depression. Patients who have a history of depression before their stroke are also likely to become depressed after a stroke. Studies show that the same medicines that help treat depression unrelated to stroke are also effective in stroke patients.

CHAPTER 11

What Are Some of the Dysfunctions, Disabilities, and Handicaps that Remain after a Stroke?

"When life gives you lemons, make lemonade."

S TROKES AFFECT DIFFERENT PORTIONS of the brain and can lead to many different types and severities of dysfunction. This chapter describes the different types of dysfunctions and disabilities, including those that

> Strokes affect different portions of the brain and can lead to many different types and severities of dysfunction.

may not be familiar to most people. Understanding these problems is an important step in overcoming or adapting to them. When there is a will, there is a way.

MOTOR DYSFUNCTION

The term *motor* refers to motion and movement of the limbs and body. Many stroke patients become weak, stiff, or uncoordinated after a stroke. The severity of weakness varies from a very minor decrease in strength to *paralysis*, which is the total inability to voluntarily move a limb or a part of a limb. Weakness usually involves the arm, hand, leg, and foot on one side of the body. This pattern of one-sided weakness is referred to as *hemiparesis* (*paresis* means "weakness," and *hemi* means "half"). Paralysis of the limbs on one side is called *hemiplegia* (*plegia* means "paralysis"). The hand and arm are usually affected more than the leg and foot. The leg most often recovers enough to allow standing and walking, but hand recovery is usually not as complete. Only one limb might be affected in some patients, or the weakness may involve the arms and legs on both sides of the body (*quadriparesis* or *quadriplegia*).

Weak or paralyzed limbs often become stiff when they begin to recover. This condition is referred to as *spasticity*. The reflexes in spastic limbs are greatly exaggerated when tested. Pressing a foot on the floor can lead to repetitive jerky movements called *clonus*. Spasticity does have some benefit, however, because support on a straight stiff leg is better than support on a leg that is loose and bends. Weight bearing is difficult on a bent, weak leg.

The arms, legs, and gait can become uncoordinated after a stroke. Patients' hands and arms may shake when trying to pick up an object. Walking can be wobbly and off-balance, similar to a person who is walking while drunk.

Motor abnormalities also often involve the structures of the mouth and throat that are involved in speaking, handling food within the mouth, and swallowing. The lips, mouth, tongue, and throat are vital in speaking. Weakness of these structures often affects pronunciation of words and phrases. Speech can become low in volume, slurred, and difficult to understand. Abnormal articulation of speech is referred to as *dysarthria*. Dysarthria is different from *dysphasia*, an abnormality of language, because the brain regions involved in production of language are very different from the motor regions that control the muscles of articulation. Very different conditions cause dysarthria and dysphasia.

Weakness of the larynx muscles makes the voice sound hoarse. Sometimes food gets caught in the throat, and the patient has to cough to get the food particles out. Most of the same muscles that control speaking are also involved in food manipulation within the mouth and throat, and in swallowing. Difficulty in swallowing is called *dysphagia*. Abnormal swallowing ability can be a significant problem for stroke patients. Good nutrition is essential to the repairing of injuries and to maintaining health. When patients cannot swallow, after a few days, a tube will be inserted through the nose and into the stomach (a *nasogastric tube*), or directly through the skin into the stomach [*percutaneous endoscopic gastrostomy* (PEG)] in order to nourish the patient. As discussed in Chapter 10, abnormal swallowing can lead to food particles and saliva and bacteria from the mouth and teeth being aspirated into the lungs, instead of food going down the correct pathway into the esophagus and stomach. Aspiration often leads to pneumonia, which can be quite serious in stroke patients, because they have difficulty coughing and clearing their lungs and bronchial structures of sputum.

As a result of the seriousness of dysphagia among stroke patients, doctors are careful to evaluate the swallowing ability of every stroke

> Doctors are careful to evaluate the swallowing ability of every stroke patient.

patient. This can be done with a simple bedside test involving the swallowing of water. At times, special physical therapists evaluate the ability to swallow using X-ray techniques that view and film materials as they are handled in the mouth, throat, and esophagus (*video-fluoroscopy*).

SENSORY DYSFUNCTION

Sensory refers to the ability to feel sensation on the limbs and body. Sensory abnormalities can include loss of feeling, abnormal sensations, or pain. Decreased feeling can affect the limbs, chest, and stomach on one side of the body. Some patients say that their sensory abnormality affects one whole side, as if a line were drawn down the middle of the body, and everything on one side feels abnormal, or less distinct. Loss of feeling often is present in the same limbs that are weak. At times, the sensory abnormality is described as crossed, meaning it affects one side of the face and the other side of the body. The loss or decrease in feeling can be quite minor; for example, not being able to tell the difference between a nickel and a dime placed in the hand. In some patients, the loss of feeling can be so severe that they cannot feel touch in an affected area. Loss of touch sensation is referred to as numbness, or *anesthesia*. Sometimes touch is preserved, but patients cannot feel painful stimulation (*analgesia*). Often the involved limbs are insensitive to temperature, and patients cannot feel hot, warm, cool, and cold on the involved limbs.

Other sensory abnormalities include tingling, prickling, pins and needles, or burning. Patients often say that the region of abnormal sensation feels as if it had "fallen asleep" after being compressed for a while. These abnormal sensations are called *paresthesias*. These sensations can be quite annoying.

Sometimes painful sensations develop in areas that are numb. Pain is usually not present in the early days and weeks after a stroke, but most often develops later. The pain may be described as icy cold, or burning, sharp, stabbing sensations. Painful feelings are often triggered by touch or use of the involved limb.

The body's sensory system can be simply thought of as having two different types of sensibilities. One type is related to coarse sensations, such as the perception of pain and temperature. Other sensations are fine and precise, and relate to touch, joint position sense, and the ability to detect vibration on the skin and bony prominences. The finer sensibilities predominate when all of the nerve pathways are intact. When these more precise sensory abilities are defective, and parts of the body are anesthetic or show reduced fine touch perception, then all stimuli seem to evoke only coarse, unpleasant sensations that often are described as very hot, very cold, or stabbing.

Pain can be compared to a malfunctioning radio. Suppose a radio is accidentally dropped into the water. At first, the radio does not work; no sound is forthcoming. The sound returns when the wires dry out, but wetting of the delicate radio wires has impaired performance, and the radio programming has become mostly static. The louder the volume is turned up, the more annoying the static. In the same way, stimulation of an anesthetic limb stirs up unpleasant feelings that become more and more intolerable with increasing stimulation. Unrecognized pressure on an arm can provoke severe pain, such as when working with the arm during therapy or while sleeping. Unlike the pain that originates from local tissues, this type of pain is "central," because it involves abnormal functioning of the central nervous system; there is no local problem in the area in which the pain is felt.

COGNITIVE AND BEHAVIORAL CHANGES

The ability to think (*cognition*) is often affected by stroke. The nature of the intellectual change can vary greatly. Loss of function can involve the creation of new memories, speaking, reading, writing, mathematical cal-

> The ability to think is often affected by stroke.

culations, and recalling where things and places are located. There can also be many types of changes in personality and actions.

LANGUAGE ABNORMALITIES

The proper use of language is extremely important for daily communication. As discussed in Chapters 5 and 7, there are different types of possible abnormal usage and understanding of language (*aphasia*). One way to categorize aphasia is to divide the possible abnormalities into motor (difficulty getting words out) and receptive (difficulty understanding what others say). The difficulty in speaking can be slight, consisting of using wrong or suboptimal words with preserved ability to get meaning across to listeners. The speech difficulty can be severe, rendering some aphasics completely mute, or able to utter only syllables or repeated single words or phrases. Sometimes aphasic patients try to get meaning and emphasis across by varying the speed, emphasis, and loudness of one word; for example, "tan ... tan... tan" or "tan tan tan tan."

Receptive aphasia implies considerable difficulty understanding spoken speech. Some patients cannot understand speech at all.

Unfortunately, most patients who have difficulty understanding what is said to them also have difficulty understanding written language, and they cannot read.

Some stroke patients lose the ability to read, but retain the ability to speak normally and to understand spoken language. Difficulty reading (*alexia*) is often combined with loss of the ability to write and spell words correctly. Loss of the ability to write is referred to as *agraphia*. Some strokes cause patients to become suddenly illiterate, meaning the patient can no longer read, write, or spell normally.

Vision (perception of written language) is handled in a different part of the brain than hearing (perception of spoken language). Alexia and aphasia can occur independently of each other, or they can occur simultaneously. Occasionally, patients lose the ability to read, but retain the ability to write normally (alexia without agraphia).

Other types of communication relate to symbols; for example, musical and arithmetic symbols. Some stroke patients lose the ability to interpret the meaning of symbols. Stroke patients may become less adept at arithmetic. They may not understand the process of adding, subtracting, and dividing, or they may understand the process but not get the answers correct. Lack of mathematical ability is referred to as *acalculia*.

Loss of Memory (Amnesia)

Memory is a complex mental function. Some stroke patients are unable to create new memories. They can hear and understand conversations, and normally engage in activities, but 10 minutes later they are unable

Memory is a complex mental function.

to recall what was said or what they did. Amnesic patients often repeat stories or conversations that occurred just a few minutes before. They ask questions repeatedly, even though the same questions have already been answered, sometimes many times. Repetitive questioning and hearing the same stories over and over can become quite tiring for caregivers and others who spend time with the patient. People become easily frustrated at continually repeating the same answers and conversations. In some patients, the inability to create new memories is temporary, lasting days, weeks, or even up to six months. In others, the memory loss is permanent.

Strokes rarely cause a loss of old memories. Some people can recall and describe vividly events from their childhood and early married years, and yet cannot recall what they did 15 minutes ago. Older memories are almost never wiped out by strokes.

Memory functions are represented on both sides of the brain within the cerebral hemispheres, but ideas, thoughts, and words are localized more on the left side. Visual memories are located more on the right side of the brain. Patients may have difficulty remembering names when the left side of the brain is injured by stroke. Remembering the names of people is affected more often than remembering the names of things. The inability to recall names is called *anomia*. This problem usually involves an inability to say the name, although usually the correct name is recognized when it is mentioned along with other names. Stroke patients may have difficulty describing objects and directions to and from various locations when the right side of the brain is involved because their visual memory is defective.

ABNORMALITIES OF INTEREST IN DAILY ACTIVITIES

Some strokes cause a decrease in initiative, and patients are not motivated to participate in normal activities. They tend to sit and do little, and caretakers may describe them as "couch potatoes." Interest in others and in their environment seems to be greatly reduced, unlike their pre-stroke behavior. Some of these *abulic* patients can be stimulated by others to go out or attend a function with them, but when left to their own initiative, they seem content to just do nothing. These same patients also become less talkative. They seldom initiate conversations, and their answers are short when they are asked questions. They have difficulty continuing conversations or giving long, detailed replies. Assembly line work involves being able to perform the same activity repeatedly. Some stroke patients cannot return to work, even simple assembly line work, because of difficulty in sustaining activity.

The opposite situation can also develop after a stroke; patients may become overactive and restless. They may become easily agitated and unable to sit or lie still. They flit from one topic in a conversation to another, and seem unable to maintain conversations, attention, or interest in any one subject or object. They exhaust themselves by overactivity. This type of patient can become so agitated that doctors call their behavior a *delirium*.

Some patients are able to continue their usual activities, but they do so more slowly than previously. Their speech is lower in volume and more often mumbled. They eat, speak, walk, and act more slowly, and it takes them longer to perform activities than before their strokes.

ABNORMALITIES IN PLANNING, JUDGMENT, AND PERFORMANCE

Some patients recover from their strokes, but do not seem to be able to function well in society despite preservation of intelligence and knowledge. In conversations, their information level is the same as before their strokes. They have no limitations in performing single acts. They score the same on standard IQ tests as they did before their strokes, yet their behavior and ability to perform is severely impaired. These types of abnormalities can be categorized as *executive dysfunctions*, meaning that these patients have difficulty planning, organizing, and performing complex behaviors.

In order to understand the nature of executive dysfunctions, it is important to review how successful people decide whether or not to do something when presented with alternatives. Consider the situation of whether or not to move into a new apartment, and which apartment among several possibilities to choose. Before acting, the careful, thoughtful individual will first examine the pluses and minuses of moving at all. They will ask the obvious questions: What are the problems and good points of their present apartment? What about the size, condition, location, cost, and upkeep of the apartment? How does it fit with the present activities and responsibilities of the individual and the fami-

146

ly? How close is it to jobs, schools, and shopping? What about safety, security, and other similar considerations? What would be better or worse in the new location? How do the other available apartments compare to the present apartment, and to the other apartments being considered? Should one of the other apartments be rented immediately, or is it worth looking further because maybe another, better apartment will come on the market?

This type of decision includes different mental functions:

- *Planning.* Before acting, thoughtful weighing of alternatives is needed. Impulsive actions may not be the best. Inhibiting instinctive impulses is important. After deciding on an action, plans need to be made as to how to carry out the action, including consideration of various possible situations that might arise.
- *Integrating various actions.* Different types of information need to be assessed and integrated before making the decision to move. This integration often means stopping one action and beginning another, and then switching again to the first activity or another activity.
- *Judgment.* Past experience, in addition to environmental information, must be weighed in order to make the decision.

Some stroke patients are unable to perform complex tasks. Cooking a meal is one example. Many factors must be considered in choosing the foods to be prepared, including health considerations, cost, availability of the desired foods, and the preferred tastes of those who will eat the meal. Then one must be sure that he has all of the needed components.

> Some stroke patients are unable to perform complex tasks.

Often, more than one part of the meal must be prepared at the same time as another. Otherwise, the food preparation might take all day, and some items will be cold when the meal is finally served. Some recipes require multiple actions and switching from one activity to another.

Stroke patients with executive dysfunction simply cannot prepare a complex meal by themselves, but these same people can help with food preparation. They can perform individual tasks when someone else directs them. They just cannot plan and integrate the functions that are needed to get the meal together.

Some stroke patients get stuck on a word or activity once started. They continue to repeat the same activity and response when they should move on to another query or behavior. This type of continuation behavior is called *perseveration*, meaning persevering inappropriately with the same response or behavior. They cannot seem to switch gears. Many complex activities require frequent switching from one activity to another and back again; for example, when asked to draw a square they are able to do so. Yet, when they are asked to make a circle, they draw another square. They may stick out their tongue when asked to do so, but then they also protrude their tongue when they are asked to raise their hands. They get stuck on the prior activity. They may also not be able to switch to a new topic of conversation, remaining stuck on the last topic.

One stroke patient said that he was afraid his mind had been seriously affected by his stroke, despite the fact that all his IQ tests were normal, and he had no paralysis or other obvious handicap. He was an executive in a large company, and customarily heard different presentations and proposals. Before his stroke he had always been able to arrive at a decision on accepting or declining a proposal, and deciding which proposal to choose. After his stroke, he found himself swayed by each proposal. He felt positive after hearing one presentation, and then felt just as positive about the next presentation. Finally, he was not able to choose between presentations. His ability to make judgments had been compromised by his stroke.

Some stroke patients become uninhibited. They do not consider the possible effects of an impulsive act. One such patient made a list of everyone who he had always wanted to tell off, including his fourth grade teacher, minister, and mother-in-law. He proceeded to visit each

Some stroke patients become uninhibited.

person and tell them what he really thought about them. Some patients become uninhibited about food intake, sex drive, or other behaviors. They act impulsively, giving in to instincts without considering the societal and personal outcomes of their behavior.

DIFFICULTY EXPRESSING AND INTERPRETING EMOTIONS

In addition to the loss of the ability to say words correctly and understand the meaning of words, which is a *linguistic* function, another aspect of communication is *nonlinguistic*. This includes the expression of the emotions and moods that accompany speech. Very different messages can be delivered, depending on the loudness, emphasis, facial expressions, cadence, and gestures that accompany the words.

Abnormalities in the nonlinguistic aspects of speech are often referred to as *dysprosody*, which literally means "abnormal speech rhythm." Depending on how a speaker says "Take the chair," the listener could conclude that she must sit down or else there will be serious consequences. Alternatively, the speaker may mean it would be nice if the listener sat down, but it is not mandatory. Happiness, anger, fear, impatience, elation, despair, frustration, and other feelings are often transmitted along with words. Reading a play and seeing the words is very different from seeing it performed on the stage by real actors.

Some stroke patients lose the ability to convey their emotions when they talk. Their speech seems flat, and they often lose the ability to pick up the emotions and moods of others. They fail to realize that their spouses are upset, angry, or frustrated. They do not detect "body language" signals. They lose the ability to tell when their spouse or significant other is tired and does not want to interact. Wishes, feelings, and moods are normally made obvious by facial expressions, tone of voice, body posture, and gestures. Detecting body signals and moods is very important in living harmoniously with others. Losing the ability to convey or detect feelings is very disabling and disconcerting to those who live and interact regularly with a stroke patient.

Some stroke patients overexpress emotions. Most often, they laugh excessively when things are not that funny, or they may cry when things are not that sad. They may laugh or cry at inappropriate stimuli, such as laughing in response to sad situations. Most of these patients have extensive motor abnormalities, especially the abnormalities that affect speech and swallowing. Exaggeration in the expression of emotions is often referred to as *pseudobulbar palsy*, because it is most common in patients whose face, head, and neck muscles have been affected by multiple strokes involving the motor functions of the muscles used in showing different emotions. Patients with this abnormality are often quite sensitive about it, and may avoid interacting with others.

VISUAL ABNORMALITIES

Many brain functions have to do with looking and seeing. Looking uses areas of the brain that stimulate eye muscles to move. Seeing is, of course, done with the eyes, but the messages are transmitted to the

> Abnormal vision is very common after stroke.

brain through different pathways. Abnormal vision is very common after stroke. The eyes are supplied with blood by the same arteries (the carotid arteries) that supply the cerebral hemispheres of the brain. Thus, blockage of the carotid arteries can cause either temporary or persistent loss of vision in one eye or a part of the eye. When the loss of vision involves a part of the eye, patients become aware of a "hole" (*scotoma*) in their vision in that eye.

When strokes affect the brain, and not the eye, they most often involve structures that relate to vision on one side of visual space. Information from the left and right eye about objects and visual information on the right side of the environment are transmitted along pathways to the visual region located in the occipital lobe of the left cerebral hemisphere. Patients become unable to see normally to their right when this pathway is damaged by stroke. This loss of half-vision is referred to as a *hemianopia*. Similarly, when the pathways in the right cerebral hemisphere are involved, patients lose their left side of vision. Some patients with a hemianopia are well aware that they cannot see to the blind side; others are unaware of the defect and bump into and miss objects on their blind side. Patients sometimes visit the doctor because of car accidents, after bumping into parked cars or objects that they could not see.

The visual pathways relating to the upper and lower regions of vision are also separated, so that some patients lose only a quarter of their vision, either the upper or lower fourth (quadrant). This type of visual defect is called a *quadrantanopia*. A patient with a left upper quadrantanopia cannot clearly see objects located in the upper part of his left visual field.

Some patients with strokes involving the right side of the brain (the right cerebral hemisphere) develop a disorder referred to as *neglect*. They do not pay any attention to objects or people located on their left side. They behave as if the left side of their world did not exist. Doctors sometimes test this by waving two hands directly in front of the patient and asking them what they see. Patients with neglect always say they see only the hand on their right side.

Visual abnormalities related to stroke can affect the complex visual functions that involve the relationships of objects in space. Some stroke patients develop difficulty in recognizing faces, even of people they know well. They also may not be able to recognize familiar places or describe objects or places. They cannot visualize in their mind the appearance of objects, people, or places. They may not be able to describe where things are located in their own rooms, houses, or neighborhoods. They may lose the ability to give directions for driving or locating specific places, and may lose the ability to read maps. Patients may become lost when they take a walk or drive a car, even in familiar neighborhoods. Artists may lose their ability to draw and copy. The size, proportions, and relationships of the objects in their drawings may become distorted and unnatural.

Some brain and motor abnormalities affect the movement of the eyes. The eyes usually work together with precision, and when one eye does not work in full cooperation with the other, patients may "see double," meaning they see two objects at the same time (*diplopia*). The objects may appear to be alongside each other, directly above each other, or angled obliquely. Sometimes, the objects seem to be moving or oscillating (*oscillopsia*) because the eyes are jiggling and moving (*nystagmus*).

URINARY, BOWEL, AND SEXUAL DYSFUNCTIONS

Inability to control the bladder or bowels is often a very unpleasant experience after a stroke. Incontinence is embarrassing for the patient, and often disturbing and upsetting to caregivers. Although everyone accepts the fact that babies cannot control their urine or bowels, somehow the same problem in adults is very difficult to tolerate, especially in our spouses, parents, and other loved ones. Sex involves the same anatomical regions of the body, and the potential of incontinence psychologically changes the sexual experience, introducing the possibility of soiling during intercourse or other sexual activity.

The nerve centers that control urination, defecation, and genital functions are located in the lower spinal cord in the sacral region. These functions occur by reflex. A full bladder creates a sensation of the need to urinate; a full bowel creates a sensation that stimulates bowel evacuation. Centers higher in the spinal cord and brain also help to control these functions.

There are collections of muscle fibers called *sphincters* within the genital region and anus. The urinary sphincters contract to hold in urine; the anal sphincters contract to hold in feces. Relaxation of these sphincters by a message from the brain allows urine and feces to be evacuated. Voluntary control of the urinary sphincters is maintained until a person reaches a location where it is appropriate to urinate or move their bowels. Control over urinary release is often affected by stroke. The reflex-induced bladder contractions become hyperactive, just as the limb reflexes are exaggerated. As a result, once the urge occurs, these patients must quickly empty their bladders or risk incontinence. Often, they cannot control or even feel the release of urine, especially when asleep. The voluntary control fibers are located on both sides of the brain. A stroke affecting one side of the brain or the descending fibers on one side usually causes only temporary loss of control of urination, because the other side will eventually assume control.

Similarly, brain centers control the anal sphincters. Normal adults can inhibit relaxation of these sphincters until they reach a suitable place to defecate. Strokes can affect the ability to control bowel release, especially if the bowels are loose. Bowel incontinence is a less common and less severe problem than urinary incontinence, because reflex functions are often sufficient to maintain bowel continence, especially with some training.

Genital sexual functions also have local spinal cord and cerebral control centers. Sexual instincts and activities are a life-long, important aspect of human life. Sex is just as important and vital after 60 as it is during youth. Strokes can seriously impair sexual functioning and inhibit normal sexual activities. The effects are multiple, and include physiologic, practical, and psychologic factors.

The entire central nervous system, including the brain, controls sexual functioning. The physiology of genital sexual reflex functions, including erection, climax, and ejaculation in men, and clitoral erection and climax in women, is controlled in the same general region of the lower spinal cord—the sacral region—as urination and defecation. These functions can be temporarily lost or diminished after strokes, but are usually not permanently affected. The brain has more to do with desire for sex (libido) and for transmission of the desire for sex to the genital organs. Libido can be lessened or increased by strokes. In some patients, the same stimuli that produced sexual stimulation and interest before the stroke may not provide the same stimulation after the stroke. These physiologic changes vary greatly, depending on the location, type, and size of the stroke.

Psychologic factors are also very important. Interest in having sex can be affected, either subconsciously or consciously, by the fear that a sexual partner might lose control of bowel or bladder function during sexual activity. Many sex partners are afraid that sex will precipitate a heart attack or another stroke in their partner. They see the stroke patient as somehow more fragile. Sex usually involves vigorous physical activity, and some sexual partners are fearful that the patient will "break." They become overprotective in every way. Of course, some spouses may not have been very interested in sex even before their partner's stroke, and will use the stroke as an excuse to decline sex. Some of the concerns and fears of stroke partners can be allayed by open discussion, although some fears are irrational and cannot be easily overcome.

Patients may be fearful and psychologically unprepared to resume sexual activity. They often fear that their performance will prove wanting, and that they will seem less of a man or less attractive as a woman

> Patients may be fearful and psychologically unprepared to resume sexual activity.

to their partners. They are sometimes fearful that sex will precipitate another stroke, heart attack, or seizure, or somehow injure them in some other way. These fears can be allayed by simply trying and accomplishing sex—in the same way that jumping in the water and swimming is the best way for children to overcome their fear of the water.

There may also be pragmatic, practical barriers to sex. Motor deficits can make positioning more complex; mobility of the trunk and limbs can be reduced. Agility in performing manual, oral, and genital stimulation may be affected. Loss of sensation after the stroke may diminish previously normal sexual arousal. Despite these difficulties, however, many stroke patients are able to resume normal or even heightened sexual activity after a stroke. Where there is a will,s there is always a way!

CHAPTER 12

How Does Recovery from Stroke Occur? How Can Recovery Be Improved? What Is Rehabilitation? Where Is It Performed and By Whom?

"To wish to become well is a part of becoming well."

Seneca

"Use strengthens, disuse debilitates."

Hippocrates

RECOVERY

THE GREAT MAJORITY of stroke patients improve; some even return to normal or near-normal functioning. Many are able to go back to

The great majority of stroke patients improve.

their previous work and resume the same activities and interests that they had before their stroke.

There are three main mechanisms that explain improvement:

- Some of the brain injury (ischemia, hemorrhage, and edema) can be reversed, and tissue injury may continue to heal for days, weeks, and even months after the stroke.
- Very few, if any, brain functions are completely localized to one place in the brain. There are reserve regions that can take over when one region is injured. This process takes time, and is clearly influenced by activity. For example, talking to and with aphasic patients clearly promotes the ability of uninjured brain regions to increase the capacity for language
- Adaptation to the deficits, that is, learning to do things in ways different from before the stroke.

The ability to return to normal functioning varies widely between individuals. There are four categories of factors that contribute to recovery:

1. Factors Related to Disease

Hemorrhage and ischemia have different mechanisms, timing, and degrees of recovery. In patients with brain hemorrhages, the blood collects between brain regions, displacing but not often destroying normal tissues within the brain. White blood cells and other cell scavengers migrate to the region of bleeding. Chemicals are discharged after hemorrhage, and very gradually the region of bleeding dissolves and is reabsorbed, leaving a slit or hole in the brain. This slit disconnects functioning areas within the brain, but usually brain regions that surround the hemorrhage are preserved. Hemorrhages are associated with more mass effect than infarcts, because extra matter (blood) is injected into the brain and skull.

It takes time to reabsorb the blood. Recall a time when you had a severe blow or fell on an arm or leg and a large bruise developed. The injury probably swelled for a few days and then the bruise gradually faded. Healing does not always happen quickly. Similarly, patients with brain hemorrhages begin to recover later than patients with brain ischemia, and the recovery period lasts longer. Recovery is often more complete in patients with hemorrhage than in patients with brain infarcts, because usually less tissue is lost in hemorrhage.

The process of recovery is different in patients with brain ischemia, because the brain injury is caused by lack of blood flow. In the minutes and hours after symptoms begin, blood flow is often restored or at least improved. Emboli that have blocked an artery can spontaneously pass and move downstream. Even when the main arteries remain blocked, other blood vessels (collateral circulation) increase blood flow to the threatened region. The brain tissue that receives insufficient blood produces chemicals that encourage ingrowth and expansion of blood vessels near the ischemic region. As discussed in Chapter 9, doctors can sometimes unblock the obstructed artery either mechanically (surgery, angioplasty/stenting, or mechanical removal of clots), or by chemically dissolving the clot (thrombolysis). In any case, improved blood flow allows recovery of some of the ischemic tissue.

When an artery is blocked, tissue fed by the artery ceases to function normally, and patients develop symptoms that indicate loss of function. There may be different severities of injury within the undersupplied area. The area with the least blood flow, usually referred to as the *core* region, has the most severe injury and is almost always permanently damaged; that is, infarcted. Areas beyond the core are often marginally deprived of blood; this tissue is often referred to as *penumbra*. When blood supply to the penumbral area improves, the nerve cells in that region regain normal function. The improvement in blood flow must develop within a few hours if brain cells are to be saved, because brain cells die quickly.

Recovery of ischemic brain tissue can occur within hours or a few days. Sometimes the degree of recovery is dramatic. Patients with total

> Recovery of ischemic brain tissue can occur within hours or a few days.

paralysis can recover complete use of their limbs, and patients who are speechless can begin to speak normally. Infarcted tissue does not recover, however. Much of the recovery in patients with ischemia occurs within hours or a few days, in contrast to recovery from hemorrhage, which may take weeks to months. Recovery is usually poor when a large portion of the brain in elderly patients is infarcted. In comparing patients who have hemorrhages and infarcts of a similar size, more brain tissue is ultimately lost in the patients with brain infarcts.

2. Factors Related to Anatomy

As emphasized throughout this book, different parts of the brain have different functions. The location of the stroke is more important than the cause in determining the types of deficits and handicaps. Vision in the right visual field is located in the left occipital lobe. A hemorrhage or infarct in this region causes persistent loss of vision in the right visual field. In contrast, an infarct in the left temporal lobe could cause a severe loss of ability to make new memories. This type of amnesia almost always goes away within 3 to 6 months, even if the infarct remains unchanged. Memory abilities are located in both temporal lobes, and injury to one causes only a temporary amnesia. Similarly, a stroke in the *caudate nucleus* on one side may cause temporary apathy that resolves, even if the infarct does not. The location of the brain injury is an important determinant of recovery.

Many functions reside in more than one brain region. When one of these areas is damaged by stroke, other regions can allow substantial improvement of the lost function. When primary speech regions in the left brain are injured, other nearby regions in the left cerebral hemisphere and some regions in the right cerebral hemisphere can subserve some of the lost language functions. Recovery by alternative brain regions is most common in children and young adults, but it is possible at any age.

Some functions, unfortunately, are located predominantly in only one brain region. Fine hand movements are controlled by the motor and sensory regions related to hand function (Figures 5-6 and 5-7). Dexterity of hand function is lost and cannot be replaced by other regions when this area is damaged by stroke.

The size of the stroke is also very important. Large infarcts and hemorrhages cause more persistent abnormalities than smaller ones.

Recovery from large infarcts and hemorrhages is delayed and usually limited.

3. Factors Related to Individual Characteristics

We all recognize that some healthy individuals are motivated, well organized, determined, and successful, while others are often characterized using opposite adjectives. The attributes, capabilities, and failings of individuals are even more important after a stroke, because they relate closely to the patient's ability to overcome adversity. Individuals who were not able to hold a job before their stroke are extremely unlikely to be successful at obtaining and keeping a job after a stroke.

Prior health conditions are also very important. Recovery from a paralysis of one side of the body (*hemiparesis*) requires considerable determination, effort, and stamina. Patients who have arthritis or prior injuries of their lower limbs will have more difficulty learning to walk again than those who had strong joints and limbs before their strokes. Prior heart and lung disease, being overweight, or being out of condition, of course, also affect the ability of individuals to generate the stamina needed for rehabilitation. Depression, which is very common after strokes, affects the will to recover.

Determination and personal strengths and abilities impact heavily on recovery. "When the going gets tough, the tough get going," is an old

> Determination and personal strengths and abilities impact heavily on recovery.

saying that applies to stroke recovery. Different people recover quite differently from the same stroke type, location, and size.

4. Factors Related to the Environment

Personal, interpersonal, social, and economic resources are extremely important in stroke recovery. The most important resource is the presence of one or more significant others who will give the stroke patient quality time, physical help, emotional support, and encouragement. It is extremely hard to go it alone when you have a handicap. Such ordinary considerations as using a car, living on one floor (especially the first floor), the presence of an elevator in an apartment building when the patient lives on an upper floor, accessible shopping, and handicap precautions and facilities can make a great deal of difference in determining what stroke patients will be able to do and accomplish. Economic resources to pay for adequate equipment and help are also very important.

Adaptation to the home setting is an important focus of rehabilitation. The home often has to be changed in order to adapt to the disabilities of the stroke patient. Installing pull bars in the shower and bath, discarding throw rugs that could result in tripping or falls, and building ramps for ready entry into the home are some examples of the types of home modifications that are often needed.

REHABILITATION

Recovery is a word that describes getting better. The focus is on the *person* or group that is injured, or in this case the individual who has had a stroke. The term *rehabilitation* has a different focus; it refers to the process of professional help in promoting recovery. Rehabilitation can take place in a special rehabilitation ward or hospital, at an outpatient facility, or at home. The choice of location depends heavily on the nature and severity of the disabilities that are present after the stroke and the facilities and personnel available in the community.

Rehabilitation Hospitals and Wards

Rehabilitation can be offered at rehabilitation hospitals, or *subacute nursing facilities* (SNFs), or at home. Unfortunately, "He who pays the piper often calls the tune," and the location is often dictated by insurance carriers. There are many differences between these types of facilities. Hospitals usually have doctors, other medical professionals, and laboratory and radiology services available 24 hours a day. Therapies are usually offered three to four hours a day, six or seven days a week. Physician availability is much less at SNFs, and therapies are usually performed only two to three hours a day, five days a week. Laboratory facilities are usually lacking in rehabilitation programs. Outpatient and home therapies have the advantage of allowing attention to adaptation to the real environment of the patient, but are limited to those individuals who have relatively minor disabilities and can be managed at home.

The personnel and programs available at rehabilitation hospitals are quite different from those found in acute care hospitals (wherein the prevailing strategy is to diagnose and treat medical illnesses). The goal of rehabilitation is to help stroke patients correct and adapt to their various handicaps in order to maximize functioning. Of course, some rehabilitation and physical therapies should be started during the initial stay at the acute care hospital. Medical care begun at the acute care facility should be continued during rehabilitation.

The first step towards remediation and adaptation to dysfunction is an accurate assessment of what the patient can and cannot do. Testing is often accomplished by a series of different professionals. This might include physicians, nurses, psychologists, physical, speech, and occupational therapists, and social workers. The doctors are often *physiatrists* (also called *physical medicine specialists*) rather than neurologists. Internal medicine specialists, geriatricians, and neurologists are often active in rehabilitation centers or available for consultation. Rarely are the doctors who provided care at the acute care hospital available during rehabilitation, unless rehabilitation takes place in a ward or other building located near the place that acute care was given.

One of the major characteristics of rehabilitation hospitals is the emphasis on a team approach, with a number of different individuals working together to identify deficits and enhance recovery. These different individuals usually begin by testing different functions. Speech therapists may test language and swallowing ability if abnormalities are suspected. Physical therapists test the strength and agility of the arms and legs, and observe the stroke patient's walk. Occupational therapists determine whether the patient can perform the common tasks of ordinary daily living and working. Neuropsychologists test thinking functions, such as memory, language, perseverance, and visual-spatial capacity. Social workers explore family, community, and financial situations and resources, so that care can be continued after discharge from the rehabilitation facility. Physicians review the medical aspects, including past and present medical illnesses, and the cause and treatment of the stroke.

Once testing is completed, there is usually a group meeting during which the patient is fully discussed and plans for management are agreed upon. Each of the individuals involved in conducting therapy then actively tries to help the patient overcome his deficits. Staff meetings are held frequently and regularly to discuss the patient's progress.

The first step toward recovery is recognition by the patient of exactly what is wrong. Education as to the nature of the potential handicap is very important. For example, many individuals who have a visual field abnormality do not recognize or understand that the problem is not in

> The first step towards recovery is recognition by the patient of exactly what is wrong.

their eye. They do not realize that their vision is limited. For example, consider Robert H., who had a left visual field defect. He had difficulty seeing and responding to objects to his left. Helping him become aware that he was not noticing objects or words on his left, and that he did not look towards the left, was the initial step in retraining his visual focus. During rehabilitation, the patient is trained to always look toward the blind side, and to make sure that they have gazed to the far outer edges of reading material, pictures, and scenes. Otherwise, they will miss objects and persons on their blind side. The education process should include the caregivers who will be with the patient when the patient returns home.

Various types of deficits are addressed by different therapists. A physical therapist may work on limb strength, exercises, and walking stability. They may help patients with paralysis learn how to transfer from bed to chair, and from chair to toilet. The therapist will show the patient how to improve function in a weak limb. Stretching of stiff limbs will be taught. The physical therapist may also show caregivers how to perform range of motion exercises, which should be continued after the patient goes home. Physical therapists will instruct the patient how to use various aids, such as canes and walkers, if needed.

Occupational therapists will review with the patient how to perform various daily activities. For example, they might work with a patient in a practice kitchen to help them regain the ability to prepare food. Occupational therapists might work with caregivers to help adapt the home according to the stroke patient's needs.

Speech therapists work with speaking, reading, and writing skills, and may also evaluate and treat swallowing problems. A number of computer programs are now available to help patients with aphasia. The speech therapist will often begin speech remediation, which will be continued in an outpatient setting after discharge from the rehabilitation hospital. They might also instruct caregivers as to the best way to manage speech difficulties at home.

Rehabilitation hospitals often have professionals who can create and fit various assistive devices, such as braces, slings, and supports. The strategy is often to correct the functions that can be corrected, but also to find alternate means of doing things that cannot be readily corrected. For example, a right-handed person who develops paralysis of the right hand will be taught to do more with the left hand. Various aids are used to facilitate hand function when an individual cannot use her hands to grasp small objects.

A very important aspect of the rehabilitation process is to educate significant others in the patient's home and environment about the nature of the various handicaps, and how they should be handled when the patient returns home. Wives, husbands, children, and other family members can help with rehabilitative therapy, and they should understand the patient's abilities and limitations.

The stay in a rehabilitation hospital may not succeed if the patient has severe disabilities. If the patient cannot go home, they are often transferred to a SNF for continued but less intensive therapy. The timing of transfer often depends on insurance coverage. The rehabilitation hospital staff may readjust the patient's recovery goals; for example, improving mobility enough so that the stroke patient can be easily assisted, rather than aiming at independence.

The process of recovery usually takes much longer than the time it took to develop the stroke, and stays in the rehabilitation hospital are usually longer than stays in the acute hospital. When patients are ready to leave rehabilitation hospitals or SNFs, it is very important that discharge planning is done to decide on further recovery strategies and outpatient therapy, if needed. Outpatient therapy can help considerably by supervising therapies aimed at strengthening, balance in walking, and fitness.

REALISTIC EXPECTATIONS

It is important to emphasize that much of the recovery from stroke happens spontaneously. The damage heals, and nature finds a way to restore some of the compromised functions. Recovery continues because of the determination of the stroke patient and their caregivers and significant others. Therapy should not be allowed to continue indefinitely. Patients

> Much of the recovery from stroke happens spontaneously.

often do not need ongoing, formal rehabilitation. Unfortunately, they are often intensely attached to their therapy and their therapists. Most physical and occupational therapists are young, active, encouraging individuals who work closely with patients. Patients improve while they are receiving therapy, and many patients automatically associate recovery with therapy. They worry that they will regress or stop improving when formal therapy is stopped; however, many patients who do not have formal therapy do get better. There comes a time when patients should stop formal therapy. After all, it takes time, effort, and financial resources, and most patients must travel to the therapy location. There comes a time when they must return to living as a person, not as a patient.

Rehabilitation therapy often targets specific functions, such as arm and hand strength and dexterity. Thus, patients will continue to vigorously work at arm and hand strengthening maneuvers, firmly wedding in their minds recovery from stroke to return of these upper limb activities. But the aim of rehabilitation is not to return all functions to normal. This may be an impossible goal. The aim is to return the individual stroke patient to as close to normal as possible. Patients can live quite normally, and do almost everything that they could do before their stroke, *without* normal hand function on one side. There are baseball pitchers and successful politicians who have only one arm. Patients should be encouraged to broaden their view of recovery toward regaining normal activities. Overemphasis on therapy and special exercises delays the return to normal activities and socialization. The individual who has had a stroke must return to thinking of themselves as a person, not just as someone who is sick. Life is short. Try to gain as much as you can from each day. Time spent on therapy and exercises is lost for other activities that you might enjoy, including movies, travel, reading, or just socializing with friends and family.

CHAPTER 13

How Does One Person's Stroke Affect Others?

"No man is an island entire of itself; every man is a piece of the continent, a part of the main. . . . any man's death diminishes me because I am involved with mankind; and therefore never send to know for whom the bell tolls; it tolls for thee."

John Donne

STROKES DO NOT JUST HAPPEN to individuals. Although only one person has had a stroke, the effect of the stroke is widespread. The family constellation and roles are often changed. The spouse or significant other now must become a caregiver in addition to previous roles and responsibilities. Children and grandchildren are affected. The stroke patient's role at his workplace may end or be altered. Community and religious organization activities are likely to change. The physical, social, psychologic, and economic burden is enormous.

THE EFFECTS ON CAREGIVERS

The caregiver's relationship with their spouse may be drastically altered after stroke. Often the caregiver, who is usually a woman, had been the more passive individual in the household in the past, and the stroke patient had been the decision maker and dominant figure. Now, the caregiver must make all of the decisions, and this unaccustomed role

> The caregiver's relationship with their spouse may be drastically altered after stroke.

may make her feel ill equipped and rather uncomfortable. On the other hand, a male caregiver may be unaccustomed to dealing with the daily household issues that had always been taken care of completely by his wife. Most caregivers are husbands or wives. They are usually around the same age as the stroke patient. They often have similar health problems and their own handicaps. Multiple new roles place enormous stress on caregivers and on interpersonal relationships with the stroke patient.

The Caregiver as Nurse

The stroke patient may require home care that is similar to care usually performed by nursing staff in the hospital. This care may include supervision of medications, and sometimes injecting medications after appropriate training. Attention to toileting and incontinence are especially stressful for some caregivers. The caregiver must often learn to ask about feelings, needs, discomforts, new symptoms, and other areas that they are not accustomed to discussing. Most caregivers have not had previous training in nursing care.

The Caregiver as Amateur Psychologist and Cheerleader

Depression is very common after stroke. Studies show that having someone to encourage, lead, push, and cajole the patient is the single most important factor in returning to the workplace and to former roles in the family and community. The caregiver must remain upbeat, even though the additional roles and stresses involved often lead to discouragement and depression. The caregiver must remain positive in the face of greater responsibility, role reversal, and stress.

At times, the stresses become so great on caregivers that they choose to leave their relationships and responsibilities. Despite the fact that the marriage vows say "in sickness and in health," illness and time often change a loved one into a totally different person from the one they married. Some significant others and family members simply cannot cope with the changes, stresses, and added responsibilities imposed by caring for a stroke patient.

The Caregiver as Therapist

Caregivers often assume roles that are normally carried out by physical, occupational, and speech therapists in rehabilitation facilities. During rehabilitation, the caregiver should be shown the exercises and activities that will be necessary when the patient returns home. This often includes how to shift from bed to chair, how to stand and walk, gait, getting on and off the toilet, and the use of eating utensils. Caregivers often need to perform full range of motion exercises to keep the patient's limbs from stiffening. Supervising the stroke patient's bathing and toileting may also require training.

The Caregiver as Amateur Physician

The patient and caregiver will be exposed to many health professionals during the stroke and recovery. Their primary care doctor or internist, the neurologist involved during the acute care hospitalization, and the rehabilitation personnel may all be different people. Unfortunately, the medical information about the stroke and its cause and management may not have been communicated as thoroughly as possible to the primary care physician, who was probably not involved during the acute hospitalization and rehabilitation. Surveys have shown that many primary care doctors and internists are not up-to-date on the diagnosis and treatment of stroke and its complications.

Of course, most caregivers are untrained medically. The brain functions and abnormalities involved in stroke are complicated and difficult to understand, and many caregivers have not been taught effectively, or have been taught and they still do not grasp the information about the brain, the stroke, and the resulting handicaps. They often do not know what to expect, what to look out for, and who to call if a problem arises. The situation is similar to that of a mother with her first newborn child. She has no training or experience in handling a helpless being who cannot communicate effectively.

The Caregiver as Pharmacist

Patients often arrive for medical appointments with a bag full of pill bottles to discuss with the doctor—often more than ten different medications! How can anyone keep all of these pills straight? Sometimes, two of the bottles contain the same substance; one with the generic name on the bottle and the other with the trade name. Questions about medications abound. When is the best time to take the pills? Which pills should not be taken together? Which need to be taken with food? Which require a period of time after use before eating? Which nonprescription pills (for example, pills for pain, colds, and sleep) should not be taken because of medical illness or because of interactions with prescription medications? The use of medicines can be complex, and all of these questions may not be easily answered by the patient's doctor or pharmacist, especially if the questions come up when professional advice is not readily available.

Pill boxes that are preloaded for the week and arranged by time of day are very helpful, but may be beyond the ability of many caregivers to use without help. Some pharmacies and personal care providers offer this service. Cleo Hutton in Appendix B (tips 13–16) offers practical advice regarding storing and dispensing medicines.

The Caregiver as Banker and Economist

Strokes clearly cost money. Salaries and money earned by the stroke patient may diminish, despite disability insurance. The caregiver may have to curtail their work hours. Medicines, transportation, and doctor visits all cost money. The bills may add up. Many caregivers, especially women, have not had previous experience with handling the money, bills, and investments of the family.

The Caregiver's Role as Spouse, Companion, and Lover

The caregiver naturally wants to continue their accustomed role with the stroke patient, but the new responsibilities and stresses may make this very difficult. As discussed in Chapter 11, there are changes in sex function after stroke. Decreased erectile function in men, and decreased sexual urge and responsiveness in both sexes are common. In addition, other handicaps, such as weakness, difficulty manipulating the body and limbs, and incontinence, may affect the ability to have sex.

Personality and behavioral changes in the stroke patient may alter interpersonal relations. Some stroke patients develop a lack of initiative; apathy; lethargy; aggressiveness; difficulty picking up body signals; voice tone, and facial expressions; difficulty speaking; depression; and other unfamiliar traits that can alter the relationship between the stroke patient and the caregiver.

MULTIPLE CAREGIVERS

The previous discussion assumes that one individual will assume the role of direct caregiver, usually when the stroke patient returns home. There may also be situations where there is more than one caregiver. This occurs most often when the stroke patient has to go to a nursing home or other chronic care facility. In this case, the spouse, significant other, or other family members will need to monitor the quality of care delivered—and hope for attention, kindness, and concern for the health and welfare of the patient by facility staff. This task usually means traveling to and from the facility at frequent intervals. Care assessment is difficult, at best.

The responsibility of caregiving can be shared among family and friends. In this case, the challenge is to divide up the responsibilities evenly and fairly, and for all of the caregivers to have similar goals. This

> The responsibility of caregiving can be shared among family and friends.

task often causes stresses on relationships that may have been tenuous before the stroke. Often, the participants have other major demands on their time and effort.

Children and Grandchildren

Children of stroke patients are, by nature, accustomed to a dependent relationship with their father or mother. After a stroke, an adolescent or young adult child may be thrust into a different role with their parent. In *Striking Back at Stroke, a Doctor–Patient Journal* (written by the present author with a colleague), the patient's oldest daughter reflected on the changes in her life that were produced by her mother's stroke. She described the strain of added responsibilities and the lack of parental guidance when she became the caregiver. The usual dependency role between parent and child had been abruptly reversed and was difficult to recapture. Doctors and nurses should emphasize to caregivers that they may need to pay even more attention to their children after a spouse's stroke. People who have children know that bringing a new baby brother or sister home is a big stress to older children, and that extra attention must be given to the older child. The family must be kept together, and spirits should be upbeat to meet the challenge. The whole family must pull together to meet the new challenges and, at the same time, continue previous roles and responsibilities.

Relationships with grandma and grandpa are often very special for children. A treasured bond may exist. Grandchildren are often devastated when a beloved grandparent has a stroke or other disabling illness. They, too, may need extra attention and explanations during the recovery period and thereafter. Often the illness or death of a grandparent is a child's first encounter with serious loss.

THE WORKPLACE

Many stroke patients had previously worked for long years in one job or for one company. The sudden absence of that individual affects the workplace. Return to work is often possible, but sometimes the tasks and responsibilities performed before the stroke cannot be continued. Flexibility at the workplace may be limited, and a change in job description to meet the stroke patient's revised capabilities may not be possible. In addition, a new job might be very difficult to find.

CHAPTER 14

What Does the Future Hold? What Research Is Being Pursued?

"Some men see things as they are and say Why? I dream things that never were and say Why not?"

George Bernard Shaw

ALTHOUGH THERE IS NO magic crystal ball that can accurately predict the future, the understanding of stroke seems to have come of age with the development of a proven treatment for stroke: thrombolysis. The United States Government, the media, the American Heart Association, the American Academy of Neurology, and the American Stroke Association have all pressed for more research and more availability of expert care for stroke patients. Clearly, there will continue to be important advances in knowledge about the various causes of stroke and treatment.

PUBLIC AND PHYSICIAN EDUCATION

Doctors cannot treat stroke patients optimally unless patients come to qualified health facilities soon after stroke symptoms develop. In order for this to happen, the public must be made aware of stroke and its manifestations. Yet, numerous surveys have shown that the public's knowl-

> The public must be made aware of stroke and its manifestations.

edge about stroke is very limited, when compared to awareness about heart disease and cancer. One of the reasons for this lack of awareness and knowledge is the complexity of stroke. The brain is much more diverse and complex than the heart. Understanding the symptoms of stroke and its effects requires knowledge of brain function. The symptoms and signs of cancer and heart disease are much simpler and easier to understand than stroke.

Children must be taught in school about the natural functions of the body. Science and mathematics education in the United States is weak, compared with Europe and some parts of Asia. Biology and health education are critical, and should be started in schools when children are young. More money and support for public education is needed. More education and information should be provided in the workplace, in the media, on the Internet, and in doctors' offices and hospitals.

The education process should extend to primary care doctors, internists, and emergency physicians. Advances in medicine and technology have developed so quickly that it has been very difficult for physicians to keep up. Sadly, many physicians are not particularly knowledgeable about the brain and stroke.

TECHNOLOGY

As discussed in Chapter 8, technology is available to quickly and safely visualize the brain and its blood vessel supply. Improvements in technology have occurred rapidly during the last decade, and further improvement is likely in the near future. However, many facilities that care for stroke patients do not have modern imaging technology readily available. In the future, more medical centers will have modern CT and MRI capabilities.

Ultrasound technology has improved even more than other brain imaging techniques, and has important advantages over CT and MRI. Diagnostic ultrasound equipment is much less expensive than CT or MRI equipment. It is portable and can be moved into emergency rooms. It can also be used in outpatient facilities and hospital wards. Testing can be repeated often, and the cost is relatively low for patients compared to

CT and MRI. Neurologists in training in some European centers are taught to use ultrasound probes so that testing can be done as part of the initial evaluation by doctors when they examine the patient. It is hoped that, in the future, ultrasound will continue to spread to more and more medical centers and stroke units.

STROKE CENTERS

In the past, hospitals were permitted to advertise as stroke centers. Many of these self-designated stroke centers would not qualify as such if they were objectively evaluated. Accurate diagnosis and treatment requires that specialized stroke centers have expert stroke care readily available 24 hours a day, 7 days a week. This capability requires doctors experienced in managing stroke, modern technology, and systems in place to ensure that stroke patients are handled quickly and effectively. Centers specializing in stroke have technology available and individuals experienced in performing and interpreting test results. Tests can and should be done quickly. Not many hospitals live up to these requirements, but most large cities have stroke centers in one or more hospitals.

The American Stroke Association and many state governments have set in motion rules for designating stroke centers. Hospitals must apply. Evaluators then check the hospital's capabilities and approve or deny the

> Undoubtedly, the number of qualified designated stroke centers will increase in the near future.

application. Primary stroke centers have adequate personnel and technology, but may not have the most advanced services. Other centers will be designated as advanced centers with complete medical and surgical capabilities, advanced up-to-date technology, and effective protocols that ensure rapid and efficient treatment of patients suspected of having stroke. Undoubtedly, the number of qualified designated stroke centers will increase in the near future.

Another predictable development will be an increase in so-called telemedicine. Using telemedicine, doctors at one hospital can consult with experts at another center. A hospital can become connected by computerized technology to one or more other medical centers. A view of the patient can be transmitted as well as diagnostic tests. This allows doctors at the referral center to interview the patient, observe, and (at times) direct the examination, and view the available X-rays and brain and vascular images. Rural hospitals and nonspecialized stroke centers can consult quickly with physicians at stroke centers for guidance. Should the patient be transferred to a stroke center? What further testing is required? What treatments should be given? Thus, management of the patient can be shared between local physicians and the stroke center. Undoubtedly, telemedicine will spread during coming decades.

STROKE SPECIALISTS AND STROKE UNITS

This book should have already convinced readers that stroke is a very complex and diverse condition. The brain is complicated, and so are the multiple diseases that involve the brain, including strokes. Advances in knowledge, technology, and treatment have developed so quickly that it is almost impossible for general physicians to keep up with modern stroke evaluation methods and treatment. Clearly, more stroke specialists are needed.

Some hospitals have specialized areas called *stroke units*. The nurses and doctors in these units have a special interest in stroke, and are trained and experienced in caring for stroke patients. The physician in charge of the unit is most often a stroke specialist. Usually, a team made up of doctors, nurses, therapists, and social workers treats and consults on stroke patients within the unit. Stroke units have proliferated in Europe. They have been shown to reduce mortality, decrease the number of patients who go to chronic-care facilities, increase the number of patients who go home, and reduce long-term disability. Everyone agrees that stroke units improve the care of stroke patients. In the future, more hospitals will develop stroke units.

NEWER TREATMENTS AND REFINEMENT OF CURRENT TREATMENTS

Modern stroke treatment is still in its adolescence. Some medications have been recently introduced, and doctors and patients are learning about the effectiveness and safety of these substances. New medications

> Modern stroke treatment is still in its adolescence.

are being developed and tried all the time. Devices have also proliferated. These devices are varied, and now include stents for opening arteries and keeping them open, retrieval devices for removing emboli from arteries, devices for closing holes within the heart, and various filters for preventing emboli from the heart and arteries from reaching the brain and other organs during procedures. In the future, more devices and medications will be developed and brought into clinical practice.

EMPHASIS ON RECOVERY

During the past decade, emphasis has been placed on prevention of stroke, and on acute urgent treatment of patients with stroke during the first few hours after the onset of symptoms. This has been very important, because it has brought stroke treatment to the forefront of the public's attention. Unfortunately, this approach will never completely solve the problem. Most patients do not arrive at medical centers with facilities for acute stroke in time for urgent treatment. Even when treatment is given in time, some residual neurologic signs often remain. The result is that many patients will survive the acute stroke, but be left with significant neurologic abnormalities.

Many diverse types of treatment can be used to help patients recover, including various medications and herbs, physical and occupational therapies, magnetic stimulation, constraint of the preserved limbs to encourage use of the weak limbs, and music, art, and speech therapies.

Most patients improve naturally after stroke. Therapy and therapists have a large placebo effect. Patients want to believe that the treatment they receive helps. Current technology makes it possible to objectively test whether a specific medication, treatment, or approach improves recovery, has little effect, or even impedes and delays recovery. We know that some medications (for example, haloperidol) significantly retard recovery from stroke. The future will include the development of further technologies, more testing of present therapies, and new treatments and approaches.

APPENDIX A

Review of
Four Patients

F OUR DIFFERENT PATIENTS were described in this book in order to illustrate the various aspects of stroke. This information appears in many different chapters, but does not include complete information about each patient. The following is a summary of these four patients.

ROBERT H.

Robert was a 68-year-old retired engineer who lived with his wife. His three children were married and were no longer living at home. He had an atherosclerotic plaque in his right internal carotid artery in his neck. When the plaque narrowed the artery, small particles broke off and caused transient ischemic attacks (TIAs). These TIAs involved both his right eye and his right cerebral hemisphere. The severe narrowing of the artery slowed blood flow and allowed a red clot to form, which totally occluded the artery. A large part of this red clot broke off and moved into his head and caused his stroke, which consisted of left limb paralysis and inattention to the left side of space.

Past History and Medical Illnesses

Robert had many health problems in the past. His blood pressure was discovered to be high 20 years ago. He had been given a number of different medications to treat his hypertension, but high blood pressure remained a problem that was not always well controlled. Ten years ago he had a heart attack and had to have heart surgery on his coronary arteries. For the past few years, he has felt pain in the right calf of his leg when he walks. His doctors told him that an artery to the leg was narrowed.

Family History

Similar blood pressure and heart problems had led to his father dying at age 51. His brother also had hypertension and had several heart attacks. One sister had a stroke.

Development of Robert's Stroke

Robert noticed that his left hand and arm felt numb one day at work, and he could not hold objects in this hand. The weakness and numbness lasted about 15 minutes. He assumed that he had leaned on the hand. Two days later, shortly after he awakened in the morning, his left face and hand felt numb and tingly for about 5 minutes. That same day, in the afternoon, a shade seemed to come over his right eye, and he could not see from the eye for about a minute. These symptoms (which were transient ischemic attacks) worried him, and he scheduled appointments with his eye doctor and primary physician. Two days later, in the morning, before he saw either doctor, he fell on the floor when he attempted to get out of bed. His wife heard him fall and rushed to him. She recognized that his left limbs did not move, but he seemed unaware of the nature of the problem. She called an ambulance and rushed him to the emergency room of the hospital.

Examination

Examination of Robert H. showed complete paralysis of his left arm, hand, and leg. He could not appreciate or localize touch or cold placed on his left side. He could not see to his left. Despite these abnormalities, when asked, he did not think anything was wrong with him. He had complete unawareness of his loss of function. He clearly had sustained severe damage to a large area on the right side of his brain.

Imaging and Other Tests

A CT scan showed a large brain infarct involving the right cerebral hemisphere. An MRA showed an occluded right internal carotid artery in his neck. A duplex ultrasound confirmed that the carotid artery was occluded. TCD showed low blood flow velocities over the right eye. An electrocardiogram showed evidence of an old heart attack, but his heart rhythm was normal.

Treatment

Robert was given the anticoagulant coumadin for six weeks to try and prevent further clots from forming in the right carotid artery and embolizing to the brain. He was also given a statin drug to deter the formation of new atherosclerotic plaques and vascular narrowing. Robert spent two months in rehabilitation learning to transfer from the bed to a chair and to walk with a cane. After several weeks, he began to recognize his deficits and became depressed. Finally, he was able to go home, but remained quite disabled by his stroke.

CLAIRE H.

Claire H. was a 29-year-old woman who lived in Boston with her family. She had a paradoxical embolus through a patent foramen ovale (PFO). A clot formed in one of her leg veins while she sat backwards in the front seat of a car on a long trip. This clot traveled to her right atrium, then through the foramen ovale during sex and into her brain, causing a stroke. The clot went into her left cerebral hemisphere, causing a loss of speech and right-sided limb weakness that improved quickly.

Past History and Medical Illnesses

Claire had always been healthy. Other than childbirth, she had never been hospitalized and had no chronic ailments. She exercised regularly.

Development of Claire's Stroke

Claire took a day trip with her husband and four young children to visit her parents in New York. It was a summer day, and the weather and car were very hot. The day was rather hectic, and they had nothing to eat or drink after 2:00 P.M. The family piled into the car at about 5:00 P.M. for the long trip back to Boston in heavy traffic. The children were restless and irritable, and squabbled nearly continuously in the back of the station wagon. Claire had to kneel on her seat in the front of the car and face backward to try and maintain safety and peace.

When they arrived home, Claire and her husband quickly put the exhausted kids to bed, had a snack and a drink, and also went to bed. Claire suddenly became unable to speak while having intercourse. Her husband realized that her right limbs had become weak, and he rushed her to the hospital. She began to move her right leg on the way there. She could talk, but did not seem to understand everything that he said. She used some wrong and nonexistent words.

Examination

Claire's speech was almost back to normal by the time she was examined. She had some slight difficulty in repeating phrases and in understanding complex questions. The strength in her limbs was normal. The reflexes were slightly greater in her right arm and leg compared to the left.

Imaging and Other Tests

An MRI scan showed a small brain infarct within the left cerebral hemisphere. Her MRA and EKG were normal. An echocardiogram showed a large *patent foramen ovale* (PFO). When air bubbles were given by vein, a considerable number of bubbles spontaneously went from the right atrium of the heart thru the PFO and into her left atrium. Even more bubbles went thru the PFO when she strained.

Treatment

Claire recovered quickly and did not require a stay in a rehabilitation facility. She did have outpatient speech therapy. Her speech improved, and all that remained to remind her of the stroke was some intermittent delay in finding the correct name for people and some objects. She was given information about antiplatelet medications and warfarin for anti-coagulation. She and her doctors chose warfarin. She met with a cardi-ologist after six months, and decided to have a procedure that would close the PFO by passing a device through her veins and into the septum between the left and right atria.

Tom M.

Tom M. was a longshoreman who did heavy physical work. He was sin-gle and lived alone. He had uncontrolled hypertension that led to hem-orrhaging into his cerebellum when he strained at work. His blood pres-sure was already high, but when he strained to lift heavy cargo, his blood pressure went even higher, causing the rupture of a small artery in his left cerebellum.

Past History and Medical Illnesses

Tom had been healthy in the past, but admitted to drinking wine rather heavily. He did not visit doctors regularly. When checked by the compa-ny doctor four years previously, he had been told that his blood pressure was "a bit high," and that it needed to be rechecked, but he did not fol-low through.

Development of Tom's Stroke

While straining to lift some heavy cargo at work, Tom became dizzy and lurched to his left. He staggered and seemed "drunk" to his co-workers. Several minutes later, he vomited and complained that he had devel-oped a bad headache in the back of his head and pain in his left neck and shoulder.

Examination

Tom's blood pressure was 200/125 when it was first taken in the emer-gency room. His pulse was regular. He was alert and his intellectual functions were normal, but his speech was slightly slurred. His vision was normal. He had no weakness or loss of sensation in his limbs. He leaned to the left when he attempted to sit or stand. He lurched in a drunken fashion to his left side when he attempted to walk. His left arm and hand were quite clumsy when attempting to reach for an object. These findings showed that his left cerebellum was not functioning normally.

Imaging and Other Tests

A CT scan showed a left cerebellar brain hemorrhage. An EKG showed evidence of enlargement of the left-sided heart muscle (*left ventricular hypertrophy*) caused by his hypertension. Blood tests were all normal.

Treatment

Tom remained alert. There was no evidence of raised pressure inside his skull, and surgical decompression was not considered. He did go to a rehabilitation hospital, where his therapists worked to improve his ability to walk. He was able to walk with confidence after several months, but still showed a tendency to veer to the left, especially when he turned. After a trial of different antihypertensive medications, three medications were found to be successful in controlling his blood pressure. He reduced his intake of alcohol.

SAM J.

Sam J. was a 73-year-old man. He had been an accountant, but was now retired. He was a widower and lived alone. His children, who lived in another city, called and visited often. He had a recent onset of atrial fibrillation. A clot had formed in his large and inefficiently contracting left heart atrium and embolized to a blood vessel supplying the left side of the brain, causing brain infarction.

Past History and Medical Illnesses

Sam had always been healthy, but recently he had noted periods when his heart did not beat regularly. Sometimes when this happened, he became slightly short of breath. He did not have hypertension or diabetes and did not smoke. He was relatively sedentary and did not want to exercise. These short bouts of fast, irregular heartbeats worried him, and he made an appointment with his doctor.

Development of Sam's Stroke

Before Sam could schedule a doctor's visit, one afternoon he suddenly realized that his right hand and leg had become weak. He felt tingling over the entire right side of his body, including his face.

Examination

When he was examined at the hospital only 90 minutes after his symptoms developed, doctors noted that his heart was beating irregularly and rapidly. His blood pressure was normal. He occasionally used wrong words and had difficulty understanding a paragraph when he tried to read. His right hand was weak, but his leg now had normal strength. He could feel touch, cold, and the vibrations of a tuning fork normally on his right and left hands, feet, and body. These findings made it clear that his problem could only be localized to the left cerebral hemisphere in an area near the lateral surface within and near the speech zone. Some of his initial neurologic symptoms had improved.

Imaging and Other Tests

An electrocardiogram showed atrial fibrillation. There was no evidence of damage to his left ventricle. An MRI scan showed a relatively small brain infarct in the area of the lateral surface of the left cerebral hemisphere. An MRA showed an occlusion of the left middle cerebral artery caused by an embolus from his heart. Blood tests were normal.

Treatment

Sam was given the thrombolytic medication, t-PA. A TCD performed after three hours showed that the previously occluded middle cerebral artery was now open. After 24 hours, he was begun on heparin and later was given warfarin.

The strength in his right arm and hand improved, but his right hand remained clumsy for fine movements. His reading remained impaired and slow.

Tips for Stroke Heroes and Those Who Care for Them

by Cleo Hutton, L.P.N.[1]

YOU ARE A STROKE HERO. Being a hero means that we continue to live with courage and commitment, and provide a role model to others. We explore new avenues of recovery while hanging on to a positive attitude. You are a hero to your family and friends. You are a hero to other stroke survivors who will face stroke head on by looking to you for advice and finding hope in your example.

TIPS ABOUT PLATEAUS IN RECOVERY

1. Choose to work at home, on your own and with the help of others, to far surpass plateaus. Many plateaus will occur during stroke recovery, and stroke heroes continually exceed them.

---

1 The 36 tips included in this chapter are excerpted from *After a Stroke: 300 Tips for Making Life Easier* (Demos Medical Publishing, 2005) by Cleo Hutton, L.P.N. They deal with the key road signs for returning home after what in some cases will have been a long route through hospitalization and rehabilitation. These tips are designed to help those who have had a stroke to achieve their maximum potential. Ms. Hutton, who has experienced stroke firsthand, is a Licensed Practical Nurse, national speaker, and advocate for stroke recovery. *After a Stroke* will complement your reading of *Stroke*, and will point you towards safety, support you through obstacles regarding emotional pitfalls, and give you step-by-step directions to plan and implement during your healing journey. You are encouraged to read the book and discover more tips for making every aspect of life fulfilling after stroke. *After a Stroke* can be ordered on-line at www.demosmedpub.com.

2. It is extremely important to have your neurologist explain to you and your family the brain areas and their functions that are affected by your particular stroke. Ask your neurologist to show you the CT or MRI scan of your stroke and explain the functions of the affected areas. Empowering you and your family with knowledge will make you better prepared for adaptive techniques.

3. If you are continuing outpatient rehabilitation, do not wait until your next session to practice what you have learned. It could be a few days or up to a week or two before your next therapy appointment. In the meantime, you and your family are in charge of practicing exercise routines taught in therapy. Brain chemical transmitters require constant stimulation in order to make new re-routed connections.

TIPS TO ASSIST READING AND COMPREHENSION

4. If you have visual defects, check with your local therapy department or local stroke support group for special techniques that will help you. Large-print material is very helpful.

5. If you own a large-print book, draw a red line down the farthest margin of the side of the page of your affected visual field. This will remind you to go back to the red line to catch the entire sentence.

6. The National Library Service (NLS) has special tape recorders to lend and books on tape that will help you in auditory learning. This service is free to those who apply and qualify. Access your local Department of Rehabilitation Services for details on how to receive this type of equipment.

TIPS ON CONTROLLING EMOTIONAL LABILITY

7. Emotional lability, a side effect of stroke, may manifest in uncharacteristic and inappropriate crying or laughing. Consult with your neurologist and neuropsychologist regarding treatment. This condition may improve in time. Shock, grief, anger, denial, and acceptance are all part of the normal emotional responses to stroke. These types of responses are not emotional lability.

TIPS FOR FREQUENT REST PERIODS

8. Alternate exercise and activity with rest periods. While you work at tolerating a longer period of wakefulness, balance it with at least one nap in the afternoon. The brain and body need more rest after stroke.

TIPS FOR ACCEPTING HELP

9. Recovery is a lifelong process that requires effort and a positive attitude. Set realistic goals. Keep a journal of your recovery process.
10. Safety is a high priority post-stroke. Accept help from family members when you move or transfer from wheelchair to chair, bed, toilet, or bathtub, especially during the first few weeks or until you can manage safely. Have a caregiver or family member observe you until you feel comfortable performing tasks by yourself.

TIPS FOR SAFETY ISSUES DURING ADAPTATIONS

11. Always wear supportive shoes with tread soles that grip well. Shoes that have Velcro™ fasteners are best. Shoes that come up high on the instep give better support and may stay on your affected foot more easily.
12. Request an evaluation of your home. A therapist can assess your needs and make specific suggestions for modifications that will simplify your daily life. Have handrails installed on both sides of stairways. A ramp may be necessary for the steps outside your home. Have grab bars installed in your shower or bath. Check that your doorways and hallways are wide enough to allow easy access for a wheelchair or walker if you use them.

TIPS FOR STORING AND DISPENSING MEDICATIONS

13. Tell your physicians, pharmacists, and dentist about all of the prescription medications and vitamins or other nonprescription medicines that you are taking.

14. Request that your medications be dispensed with bold print labels and easy flip-top lids, not childproof caps. If you have children in the home, store medication in a locked drawer and keep refrigerated medications in a locked container, too.

15. Prepare your medications at the same time every week to establish a pattern, and make sure you understand each medication's actions and side effects. Once a week, set your medications up in a plastic tray that contains spill-proof, flip-top lids. These medication containers can be purchased at drug stores or pharmacies, or obtained through your hospital. Make sure the container is clearly marked with the day of the week and time your medication should be taken. Keep them away from children.

16. When traveling, bring with you your medications and an emergency card containing your physician's name, contact number, and a list of all medications you are currently taking.

TIPS FOR DRESSING AND UNDRESSING

17. Lay out all the clothing you will wear the next day the night before. First, think of the clothing you wear next to your skin, then your socks, and lastly, your outer clothing, such as a shirt, pants, and shoes.

18. Undress your unaffected side first, and clothe your affected side first.

19. It will be easier, and much safer, to dress and undress in a sitting position, rather than trying to balance while standing.

20. If you have a leg brace, it should be fitted with a shoe with good support. The shoe needed for the foot with the brace may be a size larger than you usually wear. When you buy shoes, you may want to buy two pairs, so you will have a shoe that fits your unaffected foot and one that fits the foot with the brace. Shop at shoe outlet stores that offer two pairs for the price of one!

TIPS FOR COOKING

21. When using a recipe, gather all the needed ingredients first, and then place a pencil mark on the recipe after adding the ingredient or finishing the step. This process will help you stay on task.

22. When using a large cooking pot, fill a smaller pitcher or measuring cup with the liquid you need and pour it into the pot after it is on the range top. Never carry hot or bulky items to or from the stove!

23. Stirring a pot on the front burner of the stovetop can be easily managed by anchoring the handle of the pan against another heavier pan on the back burner. Place the handle of the first pan at the counterclockwise position against the heavier pan and stir clockwise.

TIPS FOR CARRYING THINGS

24. Use an apron or hunting vest with several pockets to carry lightweight objects.

25. When you are able to walk without a walker or cane, practice carrying things by using an empty, lightweight, unbreakable Styrofoam cup in your affected hand and walking a few steps. Gradually move up to carrying an empty paper cup, empty soft drink can, or other nonbreakable item while walking.

TIPS FOR MOBILITY

26. When shopping, use the motorized carts provided by many stores. They are usually located at the front of the store.

27. Ask your physician to authorize a disability parking permit for your car.

TIPS REGARDING RELAXATION

27. Mirrors are a very important piece of equipment in your process of recovery. Have several sizes, including a full-length mirror, at your disposal. Try facial exercises in front of the mirror. Use mirrors to help you visualize how you form words. Mirrors can also be used to view your affected side, too.

28. Music is very useful. Focus on the sound. Concentrate on the crescendos and tempo of the instruments. Relax to the rhythm of gentle music.

30. Meditation or relaxation exercises play a large part in stroke recovery. Meditation is a form of biofeedback. Relax and feel the soft beat of your heart as it pumps rhythmically. Breathe normally, pulling air in through your nostrils and out again. Picture in your mind the blood, rich in nutrients, flowing from your heart to your brain. Picture your brain using this rich fluid to nourish expanding areas. Picture the electrical impulses constantly humming in your marvelous human body. Picture your brain healing and nurturing your body.

TIPS FOR BUILDING NEW CONNECTIONS WITHIN YOUR BRAIN (SENSORY INPUT)

31. Touch every part of your affected side. Manipulate your affected fingers and hand with your unaffected hand while you are watching television, relaxing in a chair, and especially while bathing.

TIPS FOR TELEVISION PROGRAM VIEWING THAT BUILDS BRAIN POWER

32. Play along with quiz shows that highlight multiple choice answers. Try to say the first thing that pops into your mind. If you are involved in the program, you may not be self-conscious about speech difficulties. Try to trick your brain into using other avenues for retrieving information. Increased automatic reflexes are part of the stroke recovery process.

33. If you want to increase your brainpower, try to remember as many advertisements as you can between programs. Turn off the television after watching a few ads and try to recite the products being sold in as many advertisements as you can remember.

TIPS FOR FAMILY MEMBERS

34. When you visit the doctor with your stroke hero, bring written questions along that apply to you, too. Caring for someone who has

had a stroke is a big responsibility, and you also need help through the journey of recovery.

35. Stroke heroes must find their own way of accomplishing daily activities. Love is positive; on the other hand, pampering with an overabundant amount of attention and doing everything for the stroke hero stifles growth toward recovery.

36. Allow your stroke hero to be responsible for some aspects of meal planning, cooking, cleaning, laundry, parenting decisions, or family management responsibilities. Stroke heroes need to be a necessary part of the family again.

APPENDIX C

Negotiating the Insurance Maze

by Dorothy E. Northrop, MSW, ACSW and Kimberly Calder

THIS CHAPTER PROVIDES a simple, useful overview of the different kinds of insurance and lessens the chance of surprises. We hope that you will use it as a tool for financial and life planning to manage the impact of stroke on you and your family. This chapter will serve as a guide to questions that you need to ask.

A stroke brings insurance coverage into sharp focus. Most people view insurance as a necessary evil that they pay a lot of money for over a long period of time in case they will need to use it some time in the distant future. Most do not really understand how insurance works, and they are often overwhelmed by insurance language when they try to educate themselves. But, however challenging such writing may seem, you *can* understand the benefits that you are entitled to—in return for all those years you saved for a rainy day by paying insurance premiums and Social Security/FICA taxes. Of course, you will probably always wish the benefits were better. You will often be surprised by what insurance does not cover, but you will be equally surprised at just how much insurance *does* cover.

There are two broad categories of health-related insurance, one that provides income protection when you cannot work as a result of illness, and one for the payment of health care costs. Social workers at your hospital or rehabilitation center may be able to help you understand these general concepts. However, variations in coverage are huge, and you are advised to get specific information from your benefits administrator, insurance broker, and applicable state and federal agencies.

195

INCOME PROTECTION

If you or a loved one were actively employed when the stroke occurred, you should contact the employer's Human Resources Department, or the union's benefits administrator, to find out what benefits you may be entitled to. A stroke does not necessarily mean you should stop working permanently, but it is wise to understand your options. Find out whether your workplace provides either short or long-term disability plans. You should discuss filing for disability with your physician if or when you feel that the overall cost to your well-being of working outweighs its many benefits.

SHORT-TERM DISABILITY

Short-term disability plans are usually group policies offered by an employer that provide partial income replacement for a period of three months to two years. These plans are sometimes mandated by the state (often referred to as *State Disability*) and are funded through payroll deductions. Currently, New York, New Jersey, California, Rhode Island, Hawaii, and Puerto Rico have this type of mandated insurance. If your company is headquartered in a state other than the one you work in, you should make sure that the benefits quoted to you are the ones for the state in which you pay taxes.

LONG-TERM DISABILITY

Employer-sponsored long-term disability policies are sometimes paid for by employers but more often they are paid for by the employee. Such policies vary widely and you should thoroughly investigate your coverage with both human resources and the company issuing the policy. If you have purchased an individual disability policy, find out how the coverage is activated and the benefits paid. Talk with your doctor, nurse, and social worker about assisting with the inquiry, or consider legal counsel if you are having problems getting the carrier to take your inquiries seriously.

SOCIAL SECURITY

The Social Security Administration (SSA) pays three types of benefits: Social Security Retirement, which is based on having paid the required Federal Income Contribution Act (FICA) taxes as a worker and reaching retirement age; Social Security Disability Income (SSDI), which is based on having paid FICA taxes and being deemed disabled; and Supplemental Security Income (SSI), which is based on financial need regardless of what a worker has paid into the Social Security system.

SOCIAL SECURITY DISABILITY INSURANCE

You can qualify for the Social Security Disability Insurance (SSDI) program if you are a legal resident, have paid (FICA) taxes, and have worked recently and long enough.

When you are working and paying Social Security taxes, you earn credit every time you earn $920 (2005 figures) during a calendar year. You will have earned four credits for the year when you have earned $3,680. You may earn up to but not more than four credits in a year. Age at the time of application determines the number of credits needed, but if you are 31 years or older, you must have earned at least 20 credits in the 10 years immediately before you became disabled. Younger people require fewer credits, but they still need at least six.

Information about the credits required to qualify can be obtained from the Social Security Administration Administration (1-800-772-1213) or their online Disability Resource site (www.4socialsecuritydisability.com)

You should apply for benefits as soon as you can no longer work because there is a five-month waiting period from the date you are deemed disabled by the SSA before you can receive benefits. SSA will ask for names, addresses, and phone numbers for all of your doctors; dates of treatment; your work history for the past 15 years; and your most recent W-2 form. If you encounter any difficulties, have an unusual situation, or have questions that SSA cannot answer satisfactorily, the A.C.C.E.S.S. (Advocating for Chronic Conditions, Entitlements and Social Services) Program (1-888-700-7010) may be able to help.

Your family members may wish to check with Social Security to see if they are eligible for benefits as well. If so, they will be asked to provide their birth certificates and Social Security numbers. Assembling all these documents may take some time and coordination, so going through the process at the same time could make it easier for everyone.

SOCIAL SECURITY INCOME

Social Security Income (SSI) is funded through general tax revenues and is not based on work history, but rather on financial need. People who qualify for SSI usually also qualify for food stamps and the health insurance program Medicaid (see page 207).

HEALTH INSURANCE

Health insurance can be confusing. It is helpful to approach it with some basic distinctions in mind. For example, where your insurance coverage comes from is different from how it is organized. Your *source of health coverage* may be an employer plan, a union, government (for Medicare or Medicaid), your own individual policy, or a combination of these. Each of these sources of coverage has their own eligibility criteria that are mainly based on employment, age, or disability status. The source of coverage also indicates who is paying the greatest share of the covered person's health care costs. But the source of coverage is different from the *type of plan,* which controls the way the plans' members actually get their health care and how the providers of that care are paid. Members of employer plans, Medicare, Medicaid, and individual plans should know that their type of plan may be a fee-for-service plan, or some form of managed care such as an HMO, or even a hybrid of both. In this section, we will describe these sources of coverage, and types of plans, in greater depth.

FEE-FOR-SERVICE VERSUS MANAGED CARE PLANS

As health care costs have climbed in recent years, health insurers have embraced various ways of restricting, or "managing," the choices patients and doctors can make (and still be covered). Years ago, *fee-for-service* (also known as indemnity) insurance was the norm—patients used whichever doctor or other health provider they wanted, and claims were submitted to the insurer who, in turn paid the bill or reimbursed the patient. Now *managed care plans*, such as health maintenance organizations (HMOs) and their variations, are the norm for most private health plans (employer-provided and individual policies). If you are covered under a managed care plan, the choices you and your health care providers make about which services are used can greatly impact your share of the costs involved.

Managed care plans negotiate payment arrangements with selected providers. These *network* or *in-plan* providers provide a relatively comprehensive array of health services, although standards are used by the managed care organization to select hospitals, health care professionals, pharmacists, and equipment vendors for participation in their networks. Formal policies and procedures exist for ongoing quality assurance and utilization review in the provision of care to enrolled individuals. There are generally significant financial incentives for enrollees to use network providers, so enrollees are wise to take best advantage of their services when possible.

The original and most restrictive form of managed care is the *health maintenance organization* or HMO. In return for a fixed, periodic payment, HMO providers offer a range of health care services, and emphasize preventive care, including check-ups and screening tests. The HMO may have a single central facility, several branch sites, or may have an array of individual providers and facility locations that have contracted to provide service for the HMO.

Two common forms of HMO are the *staff model*, in which physicians and other providers are employees of the HMO; and the *individual practice association*, or IPA, in which physicians and other providers maintain their personal practices but agree to serve as HMO providers under the terms of the HMO when caring for an HMO enrollee.

In the traditional HMO, an enrollee who goes out-of-plan does not receive any coverage or reimbursement for those outside services, except in special cases such as emergencies. All HMO plan members must designate one physician, usually a family physician or internist, as their *primary care provider* or PCP. The PCP not only provides all of the individual's primary, or basic health and preventive care needs, but also controls the member's use of specialists. In traditional HMOs, members do not receive coverage or reimbursement for the services of specialists unless the PCP has recommended it in the form of a written referral. In effect, this puts the PCP in the role of a gatekeeper to all specialty services.

In response to consumer demand for more flexibility than traditional HMOs offered, some health plans created less restrictive forms of managed care. In preferred provider organization, or PPO arrangements, physicians and other providers contract with the PPO to reduce their fees when a member of the plan comes to them for service. Plan members may choose to use PPO network providers, or out-of-network providers. Using providers outside the network provides members some coverage, but less than if they had used one of the preferred providers. PPO members also designate a primary care provider, and will secure a higher level of coverage or reimbursement for specialty services when they obtain a written referral from their PCP, but this is not required to assure some level of coverage for a service.

Do Managed Care Plans Work Well for People Requiring More Specialized than Primary Care?

Managed care organizations work the same way for people who have had a stroke as they do for other enrollees. However, some studies and individual anecdotes raise some concerns. These concerns relate mostly to the number of specialists in managed care networks, as well as the "hassle" of the gatekeeper system. For example, the managed care networks may have very few (or no) neurologists or other health care providers who are expert in caring for people who have had a stroke. Or, they may have such specialists, but the enrollee can only receive a referral for specialty care if the primary care provider agrees to provide one. Because the managed care organization places great emphasis on saving money, the primary care physician may have major financial or other incentives to limit referrals to specialists.

Informal surveys suggest that enrollees who have adequate access to specialists are generally pleased with their managed care experience. They are usually dissatisfied with the managed care organization when they have inadequate access. PPOs try to address this problem by offering some coverage for out-of-plan consultations or treatment, but they are often more costly than HMOs.

In short, people who have had a stroke may fare well in managed care organizations if their plan is a comprehensive one and, most important, provides ready access to necessary specialists. When considering enrolling in a managed care plan, make sure to ask about access to specialists and access to neurologists.

PRIVATE HEALTH INSURANCE: GROUP AND INDIVIDUAL PLANS

At present, employers and unions may choose, but are not required, to provide health coverage as a benefit to their employees or members. If they do provide health benefits, the employer or union also decides whether dependents and retirees will be eligible for the group plan, but by law, may never exclude an eligible individual based on his/her medical history or health status. Most employees who are offered coverage as a benefit choose to accept it (by selecting among the plans offered) but are not required to do so.

EXTENDING GROUP HEALTH BENEFITS AFTER YOU STOP WORKING

Health Benefit Provisions in the Consolidated Omnibus Budget Reconciliation Act of 1985 (COBRA) are designed to ensure that people who lose employment-related group health insurance benefits for various reasons will be able to maintain group coverage for themselves and their families for a limited period. If you and other members of your family are covered under a group health plan through your employer or union that is subject to COBRA, you will each have the option to maintain coverage at a slightly higher premium for 18 to 36 months depending on the reason, or "qualifying event." However, the employer no longer contributes to the premium, and the full cost of coverage becomes the responsibility of the employee.

The law generally covers group health plans maintained by employers with twenty or more employees. It applies to plans in the private sector as well as those sponsored by state and local governments. COBRA does not apply to plans sponsored by the federal government, certain church-related organizations, or to companies with fewer than twenty employees. However, many states have *mini-COBRA* laws that provide continuation protection for those employed in businesses with less than twenty employees, although this protection is often not as generous as the federal legislation.

A COBRA plan can be terminated if the employer discontinues group health coverage, the employee-paid premium for continuation of coverage is not paid on time, the covered member becomes entitled to Medicare, or a covered member obtains coverage from another employer plan. Note that you should not drop your COBRA coverage without carefully checking the date any new coverage takes over.

Even if you qualify for Medicare, family members who are covered under your plan will qualify for COBRA coverage for 36 months. Employers and unions subject to COBRA are required to inform their members of their COBRA rights. Likewise, employees are subject to very strict deadlines for notifying the plan administrator about electing COBRA and (if applicable) the Social Security Administration's approval for disability benefits. Make sure that you understand the rules and adhere to the requirements to avoid accidentally missing a deadline and losing coverage.

Health plans that are not subject to COBRA may offer a standard conversion to another health plan. This coverage will generally be less comprehensive than the employer group plan and will likely cost more than the premium charged within the group.

INDIVIDUAL INSURANCE

Some self-employed individuals and others not eligible for group plans purchase health insurance for themselves and their dependents as individuals. As a general rule however, eligibility for individual insurance is based on one's health status, and securing coverage is not likely to be an option for stroke patients. Even when individual policies cover both an individual and his/her dependents, they are not considered group plans.

COVERAGE AMOUNTS

No matter what type of plan is used, one should always remember that having health coverage only insures your use of *covered* services—that is, services and items that are eligible for coverage under your particular contract. So long as you meet all of the policy and procedural requirements for using covered services, your plan will either pay a specific sum (a part or the total cost of your care) to your provider or reimburse some or all of your costs directly to you if you pay the provider.

The exact amount that you will be reimbursed depends on the terms of the insurance contract, but it is typically a percentage of the "usual, customary, and reasonable" cost. This cost is determined by health plans and reflects their calculation of the standard amount charged by the same type of providers for the same service in the same community. Unfortunately, many plans may restrict coverage for services or items commonly required by people who have had a stroke, such as physical therapy, wheelchairs, or homecare, particularly after the initial treatment and stabilization period.

MEDICARE

Medicare is a federal health insurance program that covers people over the age of 65 and many people with disabilities under the age of 65. If you are entitled to Social Security Retirement or SSDI benefits, you are also eligible for Medicare. People with disabilities must wait 24 months after receiving SSDI benefits to become eligible for Medicare.

Some public employees and clergy are exempt from Social Security taxes because they have paid into a separate retirement system, and thus are not eligible for Social Security benefits. However, many of these employees have paid Medicare taxes. Other individuals qualify for Social Security and Medicare through their spouse's work history.

The Medicare Program began long before managed care, and the benefits were organized very much like private insurance contracts typical of that time. These included component parts for hospital coverage, and other "major medical" services. Traditional Medicare, which covers the great majority of Medicare beneficiaries today, retains that model in the form of Parts A and B. Part A of Medicare covers hospital, qualified skilled nursing home stays, and (limited) home care. If you are eligible for Medicare, you cannot decline Part A coverage. Part B is optional and requires a monthly premium. Part B covers outpatient hospital care, doctor's fees, diagnostic tests, durable medical equipment, ambulance service, and many supplies. We recommend carrying this coverage unless you have comparable coverage from another source, as these services are used extensively by people who have had a stroke. If you choose to elect Part B, your monthly premium will be automatically deducted from your social security check.

As a fee-for-service program, traditional Medicare has many advantages. You can use any physician or certified home care agency or equipment vendor that accepts Medicare. If the provider does accept Medicare, they are required to bill Medicare directly, relieving the beneficiary of that responsibility.

Traditional Medicare's disadvantage is that it does not cover all of your costs and has not covered prescription medication. (The Medicare Modernization Act, which will offer Part D prescription drug plans, takes full effect in 2006. See page 206).

Becoming eligible for Medicare can have major consequences for any other health coverage that you have, so it is best to know what will happen to your current insurance policy *before* you become eligible for Medicare. Counseling is available through your state health insurance counseling program (SHIP). Contact Eldercare at 1-800-677-1116 if you need help locating your local program.

MEDICARE SUPPLEMENT (OR "MEDIGAP") PLANS

Medicare pays a large part of the cost of covered services, but the insured individual remains responsible for Medicare deductibles and coinsurance, and for services and provider charges not covered under Medicare. These additional costs can be substantial. To insure these unpaid costs, many private insurers offer Medicare Supplement (also called "Medigap") plans to supplement Medicare services, and this can significantly reduce beneficiaries out-of-pocket cost burden.

Initially, there was a bewildering array of Medigap plans on the market and many questionable marketing practices, such as companies selling several overlapping plans to the same individual. To address these problems, the National Association of Insurance Commissioners developed ten standardized Medigap plans, called "A," "B," "C," and so on, through plan "J." While each plan differs in the specific coverage offered, a given plan is always the same wherever it is sold in the United States. If you purchase plan F in New York, it will be identical to a plan F purchased in California, Nebraska, or elsewhere; however, it is important to note that individual companies charge different amounts for the same plan. Thus, insurance company X may charge more for plan F than insurance company Y does for an identical plan F. Medigap plans must accept all people over age 65, regardless of medical history or health status. Unfortunately, there are no federal regulations requiring insurers that sell Medigap plans to sell them to Medicare beneficiaries under age 65. Insurers that sell Medigap policies typically only offer a few of the plans at most. Your local State Health Insurance Counseling Program (SHIP) office can help tell you what is available where you live.

MANAGED CARE OPTIONS FOR MEDICARE BENEFICIARIES

Some Medicare recipients will opt for a *managed Medicare* plan, Plan C, instead of traditional Medicare. In these arrangements, all the benefits of Medicare A and B, and often some additional benefits as well, are bundled together under one plan. While the Medicare HMOs and PPOs offer "one stop shopping," it is important for beneficiaries to be aware that when signing on for managed Medicare, you are signing over your long awaited Medicare benefits to a private insurance company to manage. Enrollees are required to follow all the rules of the HMO/PPO to get coverage for health care costs (see description of HMO and PPO plans on pages 198–201.), but the plan must cover at least everything that Medicare A and B covers. Enrollees in Medicare managed care plans do not purchase Medigap policies, because it would duplicate benefits already provided by the HMO or PPO.

COORDINATING MEDICARE WITH OTHER COVERAGE

If you become eligible for Medicare due to a disability, you may or may not be able to maintain other private coverage that you already have from an individual, or spouse's policy. Even though there may be a substantial premium cost involved, many people find it beneficial in the long run to continue this coverage, as it may be more comprehensive in terms of benefits and provide more generous prescription drug plan benefits. You should check with the health plan administrator of your private policy to see how they *coordinate benefits* with Medicare. Make sure you understand which policy is *primary*—meaning it is billed first—and how benefits are coordinated between the two.

When you are covered by more than one type of insurance that covers the same health care expenses, one pays its benefits in full as the primary payer and the other pays a reduced benefit as a secondary or third payer. When the primary payer does not cover a particular service (such as medications or certain types of equipment) but the secondary payer does, the secondary payer will pay up to its benefit limit as if it were the primary payer.

Before you make a decision to keep or terminate your private coverage when your eligibility for Medicare begins, contact your SHIP for more consultation about the decision and coordination of benefits between your individual or group coverage and Medicare.

MEDICARE PRESCRIPTION DRUG PLANS

Beginning in 2006, new Medicare-sponsored prescription drug coverage will be available for purchase to help with the cost of prescription drugs. Note that those who already have prescription drug coverage that is the same or better than what Medicare will offer will not benefit from having this additional coverage, so they should not make any changes. Those Medicare beneficiaries who do want the coverage will have a choice between a "stand alone" prescription drug policy (known as Part D), or a Medicare managed care plan, including prescription drugs (known as Medicare Advantage plans). The costs involved are significant, and substantial federal subsidies are available for those who qualify for them. People who buy a Part D plan will pay a monthly premium. They will be responsible for an annual $250 deductible and 25% of costs between $251 and $2,250. Once their covered drug costs exceed that amount, they will be responsible for 100% of costs between $2,250 and $5,100, at which time catastrophic coverage kicks in—Medicare pays 95% of covered drug costs, the beneficiary pays the remaining 5%.

MEDICAID

Medicaid is a medical assistance program for certain individuals and families with low incomes and assets. In addition to comprehensive hospital, medical, and prescription drug coverage, Medicaid also pays for an array of long-term care services, including nursing home stays. Many people find they are ineligible for Medicaid, because their family income and assets are too high, or they do not meet other criteria.

Medicaid is a joint program of the federal government and each state. The federal government shares the costs of Medicaid with state governments, and mandates coverage of certain benefits as a minimum. States determine the eligibility criteria and select which (if any) additional benefits to include for their residents. Thus, it is important to know about the eligibility criteria and benefits package of your state's Medicaid program. Note that some state Medicaid programs give special consideration in their eligibility rules for people with very high ongoing medical bills known as "spend-down."

VETERAN'S ADMINISTRATION (VA)

Every veteran could benefit from contacting the VA to learn if she is eligible for any benefits (1-800-827-1000). If you qualify for medical or disability benefits, they could be an important way of supplementing Medicare, including prescription drug coverage. If eligible, you should make an appointment with a VA primary care physician and ask for referrals to a neurologist *and* a physiatrist (rehabilitation doctor) to maximize your access to rehabilitation benefits.

LONG-TERM CARE POLICIES

Long-term care policies are being purchased with greater frequency. They are designed to provide benefits that are not traditionally covered in regular health care plans. Typically, they will pay for custodial or attendant care in the home or in an outside facility.

Most of these policies have a waiting period during which you are expected to cover the cost of care for a period of time—three to six months is common. Many of these policies include some coverage for equipment. There may be services or items you need that regular insurance does not pay for that could be covered under this policy.

Benefits from a long-term care insurance policy are likely to be available only to those who have a policy in effect at the time of their stroke. Once a stroke has occurred, obtaining such a policy will be extremely difficult.

THE FINAL WORD, EXERCISE YOUR RIGHT TO APPEAL

At times, you will find that your insurance does not pay for things that you think it should. Every health plan member has the legal right to appeal a plan's decision that is not in the member's favor. All health plans must provide a written Explanation of Benefits (EOB) describing what has been covered or denied, including details on partial coverage. Check the list of Covered and Excluded Benefits in your plan manual to see if the service or item is listed under either category. Review the EOB carefully to assure you understand the plan's rationale for denying or limiting the benefit. If you and the health care provider who prescribed the service or item believe the plan is in error, follow the plan's procedures for filing an appeal. This is easier than many people and their doctors realize, although timeframes for pursuing an appeal must be observed. Your providers written support for the appeal is not always required, but it is often the strongest part of an effective appeal.

It seems unfair that when you need to concentrate on maintaining your health, so often your health plan feels like an adversary. Let your employer know if you feel that your insurance company is being unreasonable. They have an interest in your receiving what they invested in the plan. Do not be afraid to ask questions, disagree with decisions, and ask for help. Often, someone you know will be willing to take on the plan with you, such as your health care team. Let them know you need their help.

Glossary

Adventitia: The outer layer of an artery.

Angioplasty: Mechanically dilating an artery with an instrument.

Anticoagulants: Substances that reduce the tendency of blood to clot.

Antiplatelet Substances: Substances that reduce the tendency of blood platelets to stick together, to stick to the lining of blood vessels, and to secrete substances that induce blood clotting.

Aorta: The large artery that extends directly from the heart and travels down the back, giving off major branches to the head, chest, abdomen, and limbs. It is the largest and most important artery in the body.

Aortic Valve: The heart valve that separates the left ventricle of the heart from the aorta. When it opens it allows blood pumped by the heart to go into the aorta. Closure prevents reflux back into the heart.

Arachnoid: A spidery membrane that surrounds the brain and spinal cord. It is the middle of three membranes called the *meninges*. It lies outside of the pia mater and inside of the dura mater.

Arteriosclerosis/Atherosclerosis: Degenerative changes in the arteries of the body that lead to stiffening, plaque formation, and narrowing of the arteries.

Arteries: Thick-walled blood vessels that bring blood from the heart to the various organs.

> **Anterior Cerebral Arteries:** Paired branches of the internal carotid arteries within the head. They supply mostly the medial portion of the frontal and parietal lobes.

> **Basilar Artery:** A midline artery in the back of the head formed from the junction of the two vertebral arteries within the head. It supplies a major portion of the brainstem.

Carotid Arteries: Large arteries that form in the front of the neck on both sides as the common carotid arteries. Within the neck, they divide at the carotid bifurcation into external carotid arteries that supply mostly the face and structures within the face, such as the nose and mouth, and the internal carotid arteries that supply the eyes and the front portion of the brain on both sides.

Coronary Arteries: The arteries that supply the heart with blood.

Innominate Artery (the first large branch of the aorta): Divides into a right subclavian artery that supplies the right arm and the right common carotid artery.

Middle Cerebral Arteries: The largest branches of the internal carotid arteries within the head. They supply most of the lateral surfaces of the cerebral hemispheres and much of the deep portions of the hemispheres.

Penetrating Arteries: Small arteries that emerge from larger arteries within the head and course at right angles into the deeper portions of the cerebral hemispheres and brainstem.

Posterior Cerebral Arteries: Paired arteries that form at the terminal end of the basilar artery. They travel around the upper brainstem and supply the occipital and medial temporal lobes on each side.

Pulmonary Arteries: The arteries that supply the lungs with blood.

Subclavian Arteries: Arteries that run under the clavicle to supply the upper limbs. The right subclavian artery arises from the innominate artery. The left subclavian artery arises directly from the aorta.

Vertebral Arteries: Paired arteries that arise from the subclavian arteries on each side. They course in the back of the neck within the vertebral column to enter the back of the head. They supply a portion of the cerebellum and the lowest portion of the brainstem, the medulla oblongata.

Atheromatous Plaque: A flat or protruding bulge in the lining of an artery caused by a degenerative process called atherosclerosis.

Atria: The two upper chambers of the heart.

Brainstem: The portion of the brain that connects the cerebral hemispheres above and the spinal cord below. It contains the nerve cells that supply the head and neck structures, and is a pathway through which fibers pass from the brain to the spinal cord, and from the limbs through the spinal cord to the brain. The portions of the brainstem are called (from below upward) *medulla oblongata, pons, midbrain,* and *thalamus.*

Capillaries: Tiny, thin-walled blood vessels that bring blood into the tissues of the body.

Cavernous Angioma: A malformation within the nervous system made of capillaries and enclosed in a capsule.

Cerebellum: The portion of the brain located in the back of the head that is attached to the brainstem. It controls coordination of movements of the limbs and eyes, walking, and speech.

Cerebrum (cerebral hemispheres): The largest portion of the brain, consisting of two halves (the left and right cerebral hemispheres).

Coagulation: The process of blood clotting.

Collateral Circulation: Blood flow that is recruited to supply ischemic tissue.

Core (of a brain infarct; the central part of an infarct): The portion that is most vulnerable to blockage of the artery that supplies it.

Developmental venous anomaly (DVA): Abnormal veins that develop because normal venous drainage is lacking.

Dissection: A tear within the wall of an artery

Dura Mater: The firm, outermost layer of the meninges, the membranes that surround the brain and spinal cord.

Dural Venous Sinuses: Large veins located within the dura mater, outside of the brain.

Embolism: The process of a particle, often a blood clot, breaking off from its source and traveling to a recipient site distant from its origin.

Endarterectomy: Removing the inner core of a diseased artery.

Endocardium: The inner lining of the heart and heart valves.

Endocarditis: Infection of the lining of a heart valve or of the heart.

Epidural Hemorrhage: Bleeding between the dura mater and the skull.

Fibrinogen (Fibrin): A protein in the blood that is converted to fibrin, a component of blood clots and of arterial plaques.

Fibromuscular dysplasia (FMD): An abnormal condition that causes thickening of arteries because of an increase in the connective tissue within the arterial walls.

Hemophilia: A hereditary blood condition caused by a deficiency of Factor VII.

Hemorrhage: Significant bleeding from a blood vessel.

Heparin: An anticoagulant administered by vein or under the skin.

Homocysteine: A normal protein within the blood. An increase in the level of homocysteine can predispose to strokes. Elevations can be due to hereditary factors or can develop when levels of vitamins B_{12} or folic acid are abnormally low.

Hyperlipidemia: An abnormally high level of blood lipids (fats).

Hypoperfusion: A decrease in the need for blood supply.

Infarction: Death of tissue caused by a lack of blood flow. (The dead tissue is called an *infarct*.)

Intima: The inner lining of arteries.

Ischemia: Lack of blood flow.

Lumen: Hole within a blood vessel.

Media: The middle coat of arteries made of connective tissue and muscle.

Meninges: The membranes that coat the outside of the brain and spinal cord. They consist of three layers (from inside out) the pia mater, arachnoid, and dura mater.

Mitral Valve: The valve that separates the left atrium from the left ventricle.

Myocardial Infarction (MI): Death of heart tissue caused by a lack of blood flow; usually due to blockage of a coronary artery.

Myocardium: The muscle tissue of the heart.

Neuropsychologists: Professionals who test the thinking and behavior of individuals using a battery of tests.

Patent Foramen Ovale: A persistence of the oval window that connects the left and right atria in utero.

Penumbra: Ischemic brain that is not yet infarcted.

Perfusion: Supply of tissue with oxygen and energy.

Pia Mater: The most inner membrane of the meninges.

Pulmonary circulation: The blood supply to and from the lungs.

Pulmonary Valve: The valve between the right ventricle of the heart and the pulmonary artery.

Rehabilitation: The process of restoring a patient back to their previous function.

Reperfusion: Restoring blood flow that had been deficient.

Secondary Prevention (prevention after an event): Measures to prevent a second or subsequent stroke.

Subarachnoid Hemorrhage: Bleeding into the space between the pia mater and the arachnoid membranes around the brain.

Subdural Hemorrhage: Hemorrhage under the dura mater, but outside of the brain.

Stent: A mechanical device for opening arteries and keeping them open.

Systemic Circulation: Blood supply to the various organs of the body, except the lungs.

Telangiectasis: Small abnormal capillaries separated by brain tissue.

Thrombosis: The process of formation of a blood clot.

Thrombolysis: Dissolution of a blood clot.

Transient Ischemic Attack (TIA): Temporary lack of blood flow causing neurologic symptoms that return to normal within a short period of time, usually within one hour. Some TIAs last longer, but rarely exceed a day.

Tricuspid Valve: A three-part valve that separates the right atrium of the heart from the right ventricle.

Veins: Relatively thin-walled blood vessels that bring blood from the tissues back to the heart.

Venous Varix: An abnormally dilated vein.

Ventricles: Structures within the brain that contain spinal fluid. There are four ventricles; a lateral ventricle within each cerebral hemisphere and a third and fourth ventricle. The *aqueduct of Sylvius* connects the third and fourth ventricles. The term also describes the muscular chambers of the heart that pump blood into the aorta and pulmonary arteries.

Warfarin: An orally administered anticoagulant.

Suggested Reading

Berquist W, McLean R, Kobylinski BA. *Stroke Survivors.* San Francisco: Josey-Bass Publishers, 1994.

Bruenn HG. Clinical notes on the illness and death of President Franklin D. Roosevelt. *Ann Int Med* 1970; 72:579–591.

Caplan LR. *Caplan's Stroke: A Clinical Approach*, 3rd Ed., Boston: Butterworth Heinemann, 2000.

Fields WS, Lemak NA. *A History of Stroke: Its Recognition and Treatment.* New York: Oxford University Press, 1989.

Friedlander, WJ. About three old men: an inquiry into how cerebral atherosclerosis has altered world politics. *Stroke* 1972; 3:467–473.

Furie KL, Kelly PJ. *Handbook of Stroke Prevention in Clinical Practice.* Totowa, New Jersey: Humana Press, 2004.

Goldszmidt A, Caplan LR. *Stroke Essentials.* Royal Oaks, Michigan: Physicians Press, 2003.

Gordon NF. *Stroke: Your Complete Exercise Guide.* Champagne, Illinois: Human Kinetics, 1993.

Hachinski V, Hachinski L. *Stroke: A Comprehensive Guide to "Brain Attack."* Buffalo, New York: Firefly Books, 2003.

Hodgins E. *Episode: Report on the Accident Inside My Skull.* New York: Atheneum, 1964.

Hutton C. *After a Stroke: 300 Tips for Making Life Easier.* New York: Demos Medical Publishing, 2005.

Hutton C, Caplan LR. *Striking Back at Stroke: A Doctor–Patient Journal.* New York, Dana Press, 2003.

Ozer MN. *Management of Persons with Chronic Neurologic Illness.* Boston: Butterworth-Heinemann, 2000.

Ozer MN, Materson RS, Caplan LR. *Management of Persons with Stroke.* St Louis, Mosby, 1994.

Shimberg EF. *Strokes: What Families Should Know.* New York: Ballantine Books, 1990.

Index

Note: Boldface numbers indicate illustrations; italic *t* indicates a table.